YOGA FOR DRAGON RIDERS

BY KATRINA HOKULE'A ARIEL

A Training Manual for Those with Inquisitive Minds and Fiery Spirits

***Also Good for Adventurers, Dancers, Internet Enthusiasts,
and Human Beings in General.***

Empower Yourself! Play in the Profound.

ArtPrana Publishing

Copyright © 2012 by Katrina Hokule'a Ariel

ISBN   978-0-9879923-0-7

Edited by Juliette Looye
Design by Katrina Hokule'a Ariel with help from Molly Mollusk
Main Photography by Natalie Anfield - www.studiofive-o.com
Ocean and tree photos by Casey Kaldal
Inside Illustrations by Jerome Chris Marcial - www.marcial-arts.daportfolio.com
Cover Illustration by Liiga Smilshkalne - www.liiga.deviantart.com

First Edition

Disclaimer: This book contains information intended to enhance wellbeing and happiness. All information is offered as-is, and is used at the sole discretion of the reader who assumes all risks from using the information provided herein. The guidance of an experienced and qualified yoga teacher is highly encouraged. Before beginning a yoga practice, consult with a qualified professional in regards to any health or physical concerns.

You are responsible for your own choices. Make good ones.

May all beings be happy.
May all beings be free.
May your path be blessed.
May your heart song be clear and joyful!

www.YogaForDragonRiders.com

This book is dedicated to:

Seekers of Truth,
Dancers of Dreams,
Lovers and Lightworkers,
All who follow the song of their heart,

And of course . . .

The Dragons!

To the trees,
To the mountains,
To Earth, Air, Fire, Water, and Akasha…

Thank you for the beauty.

With a humble bow and deep gratitude to all of my teachers, human and otherwise.

FIND YOUR PURPOSE.

LEARN. LOVE. PLAY.

AWAKEN AND DELIGHT.

Table of Contents

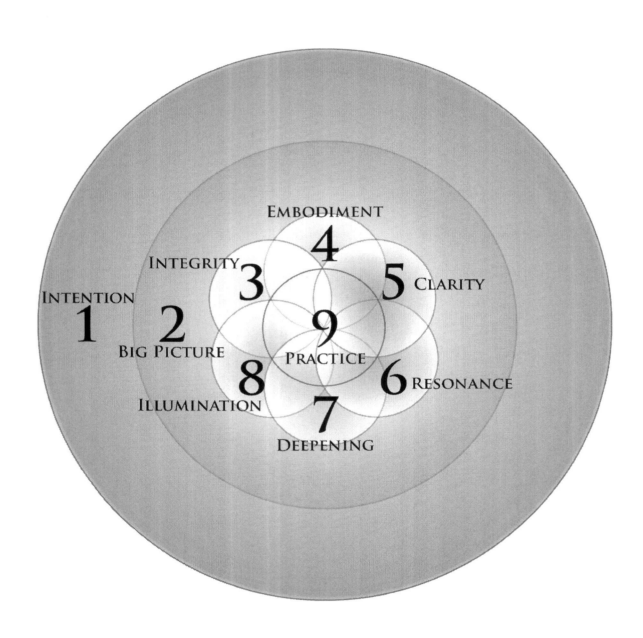

Introduction

The Call of the Heart

"You are chosen because you have asked."

Greetings!

You know why you are here. If you are reading these words, you have been called.

You have asked the deep questions of the heart and aspire to awaken to a more fulfilling, enriching, and meaningful life.

Your path is one that has wandered and wound its way through many challenges, and you have survived, grown, and evolved to become who you are today.

Your heart desires the magic you know exists, but you have yet to fully understand how completely this magic actually surrounds you, even in the seemingly dull and mundane of that-which-must-be-done.

You yearn for the extraordinary and know that you have unique talents and capabilities, even if you are not fully aware of what they are.

This is an Invitation.

If you wish, you can take this Rider's Training Manual and begin a series of Initiations that will make your path through life far more clear and resplendent!

But know this: it is not an easy path. It will come with difficulty as well as delight.

Is it worth it? Absolutely!

Your capacity is great; discover how great! Become who you want to be, taking on the virtues of those you admire and making them uniquely your own.

Ride the waves of life.

Unleash your inner Dragon.

What Is Yoga For Dragon Riders?

Yoga for Dragon Riders is a way of tapping into a wealth of wisdom and power with the guiding force of love, expanding the delight of life in service to the highest.

Yoga is the scientific art of bringing the Universal and Individual aspects of who you are into a state of conscious and joyful union.

It encompasses physical, mental, emotional and philosophical practices that transform the practitioner like alchemy—refining and revealing the sparkling essence of who you are.

Yoga is the method by which Dragon Riders and Seekers of Truth emerge from where they are hidden, deep within, sleeping beneath the limiting ideas of human habits and conditioning.

Yoga is ancient, with many secrets to be uncovered, and yet it has evolved to become one of the most liberating approaches to live a life filled with meaning—a life where laughter and silence are equally revered.

This particular approach to yoga invites your imagination to swirl and play, informed by many Masters who have passed their knowledge to me, and seen through the lens of my own interpretation of yoga. I also have infused much wisdom from other spiritual explorations, as well as journeys in the Akashic Records and the Library of Life.

This approach to yoga invites you to find your own path and creative expression, guided by principles and practices that are effective and empowering, playful and profound.

And what is a Dragon Rider, exactly?

In the context of this book, a Dragon Rider is one who lives life fully, walking his (or her) own path with integrity, honor, and skill—one who discovers what it is to have balance between the essential elements of love, power, and wisdom.

A Dragon Rider is one who connects with the power of life and the spirit of dreams—one who explores on many planes of existence, with one foot in this world and one in the next.

A Dragon Rider goes beyond limiting ideas to explore who they are, with creativity and delight, contributing their own unique talents to help uplift the world.

We can use the word Rider, or we can use the word Yogi, or perhaps the title Master-in-Training. Whatever you prefer is fine.

I like the word Rider because the idea of riding a Dragon infuses a sense of power and destiny that calls the imagination to awaken and participate more fully in your experience of life. This image invokes and magnifies the delight of creativity and therefore the force of transformation.

I also often compare life to an ocean, and we are constantly riding the waves of life.

To ride skillfully, or to surf these waves, requires proficiency and willingness. When you have both, you can find beauty and benefit both in the low times and the high times and can balance yourself wherever you are and whatever you experience.

To be a Rider (to live your yoga) is to realize that the energy that pulsates within your blood and breath is the same energy that moves the waves and is the water.

This energy is all of life, all of what you see and do not see.

And it is sentient. Aware of itself and limitless in power and possibility.

To be a Dragon Rider is to align with this energy, with love and respect: to spread your wings and fly upon the current of Grace.

Dragons remind us that magic is real, and that it exists within us.

Your Dragon is a guide and companion that may or may not manifest on this plane of reality, but is, nonetheless, entirely real.

Dragons have long symbolized power and transformation. Now, as the world changes, we must choose how to create the new world and the next Great Age of the Earth.

Dragons, along with a host of other beings both ancient and wise, have chosen to participate. They have decided to influence and illuminate this shift, so that we may finally enter the long awaited Golden Age.

Who Am I?

I am who I am.
I share what I have to offer.

If it's for you, take it.
If not, may your path be blessed.

Once I did not know who I was. Once I was lost and desperately seeking answers, comfort, and clarity. But, no matter how many times I stumbled or dug myself into holes of doubt, I did not give up.

I continued to seek magic and light until I became them!

My name is Katrina Hokule'a Ariel.

Hokule'a, my star name, is Hawaiian and means "Star of Gladness."

I am Earth-healer, daughter-of-joy and star-child-of-light.

I am sage-song-weaver.

I am the culmination of who I have been (warrior, queen, clan mother, chief's daughter, and many more besides), and I am more than all of these combined.

One of the many names my Dragon uses is Seeker of Truth.

My name has changed as I have changed, just as who you are is changing right now.

My soul's mission is to be a bright, balanced light in this world, to enjoy myself and life fully as a being of love, and to bring to others happiness and hope.

I am joyfully committed to helping this magnificent Earth come into a place of harmony; befriending trees, animals, and people alike; and calling all hearts and beings to their highest purpose with an invitation to celebrate and connect more deeply than ever before.

My own teachers are Masters from this world and also from beyond this world. I read the records of the Akasha, and in doing so I delve into the essence of What Is, for every thought, sound, and action leaves an impression in the field of energy.

It has become my dharma (my duty

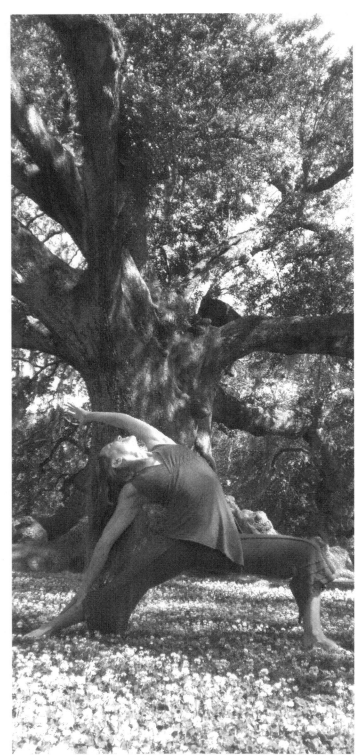

and purpose) to share the teachings I have been given, from sources both human and otherwise, for the highest good of all.

Here is one such teaching, a Great Truth in its own right:

> *Believe in yourself. Believe in the magnitude of your power, of which you feel but a fraction. Be whole, both in your vision of yourself and the world.*
>
> *You can create anything you want; truly you are capable of ANYTHING! But you must hone your skills in order to do so with Grace and clear intention. Be unafraid, you will be well guided along your path.*

What you can expect from me...

You can expect me to be straightforward with you.

I am honest, and I have learned many things from many teachers, in this world and beyond, that apply directly to our everyday lives.

Everything in this book is a real teaching. I use the illustration and symbol of Dragon and Rider as a theme to present practices, philosophies, principles, and paradigms—all of which are real and available if we know how to align and perceive.

I share my voice, my perspective, and a wide variety of information from many sources.

I teach from the heart.

I invite you to be open-minded and adventurous as you take this journey.

Explore in the realm of infinite possibility.

Take what calls to your heart and live it.

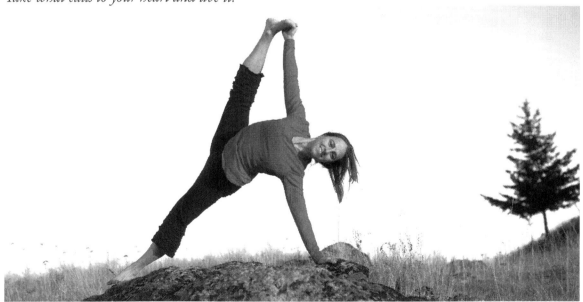

In order to skillfully become a Dragon Rider, you must be many things:

Your mind must learn to be sharp yet spacious, focused yet flexible, and able to truly perceive what is possible beyond the commonly accepted paradigm of everyday life.

Your body must become strong yet sensitive, your movements deliberate and daring, and your actions must be informed by an awareness of how all things are interconnected.

You must be willing to truly acknowledge and accept the wisdom and evolution of your spirit.

You must be able to listen, truly listen, to the song of your heart.

And you must be guided by Empowering Principles of Integrity that allow you to know exactly what to do, even when faced with fear and uncertainty.

You can learn this.

You can experience the incredible joy, exhilarating power, and tremendous freedom that come from skillfully serving the highest within yourself and in all the world around you.

This is a practice for seekers from all races and ages of the world. It asks you to deepen your faith in yourself, and the Truth you already know deep within your heart, becoming ever more empowered and inspired by this practice.

This is a path of high honor. It requires courage, yet it is infinitely rewarding.

The question is, are you willing?

Are you a Seeker of Truth and Beauty?

Are you a Warrior of Peace, willing to do the work necessary to create harmony within and without?

Do you have what it takes to be a Dragon Rider? Do you have the imagination to look beyond limiting thoughts and ideas, the determination to move towards Mastery moment by moment, and the curiosity necessary to uncover the secrets of living life to its fullest?

With great power comes great responsibility. Know this.

Know that if you choose to enter into the Rider's Realm, you will be rewarded with the soaring brilliance of liberation. You will illuminate mind, body, and spirit. And you will take a journey to claim your power with integrity while serving the highest good with courage and honor.

For a new age is upon us, and Riders of great skill and capability are needed.

If, with full knowledge of both the requirements and responsibility, you choose to accept this invitation, then we are well met. Well met indeed!

Feel free to write notes and draw all over the margins...

About This Book

This book is intended to be a joyful, radical exploration into yoga and beyond.

Think of yourself as a Dragon Rider. You immediately imagine yourself as a more powerful being. You see yourself in a new way, supported by a mighty Dragon, and access aspects of yourself that may otherwise remain hidden.

To claim your power is to embrace your entire self, as well as the mission or purpose of your life.

This must, of course, be supported by a solid philosophical and ethical foundation that allows you to be powerful in a balanced, harmonious way.

Your intent and vision must be pure.

> *I am pure. The purest of the pure.*
> *I accept my power, I embrace my power, I claim my power.*
> *For there is only Light to wield!*

By positioning your thoughts to consider yourself a Dragon Rider, you engage the immense might of your imagination and expand your ideas about yourself. You begin to dissolve the boundaries of thinking that trap you in a limited view and experience.

The world we live in is far more than we think. We see only a fraction of the spectrum of light that reaches our eyes and process only a small amount of the information that filters in.

The Third Dimension, this plane of existence that we consider the real world, is only one level of what is truly available.

By going beyond limiting ideas and practicing methods that refine and hone your skill as a being of great worth and capability, this book invites you to live fully in the Third Dimension, and to move towards the higher dimensions, where anything is possible.

In order to do this we make small, incremental shifts in the way we relate to ourselves and the world around us and formulate our thoughts in clear, deliberate ways.

Thoughts become things, and as you journey toward higher dimensions, your thoughts manifest immediately! Best, then, to be very skilled with how you direct your thoughts.

The methods of yoga and energy work presented in this book are very real and very effective.

Though approaching these practices from the concept of becoming a Dragon Rider is somewhat different, it serves the purpose of allowing you a bigger picture of yourself and what is possible. This will speed up your progress as you practice, because it is our own limiting beliefs that, so often, hold us back.

Merging Fantasy and Reality

I often describe myself as part cat, part elf, and part hobbit . . .

When I was a little girl, I yearned for a world filled with magic and wonder. That desire never left me, and so I fulfilled it by diving into books of fantasy and adventure.

For a long time, I wished so many of the elements of those books could be real. Then, through my explorations in yoga, meditation, energy, philosophy, and discoveries that most history books don't tell you about, I realized that those elements ARE real.

If you take every fantasy book and look at the common characters and concepts, there are threads that stand out and weave the many worlds together.

These commonalities are all reflected in who we are and the world around us, if we but look.

THE ELEMENTS OF THE EXTRAORDINARY

1. The conflict of good and evil:

Every fantasy book is a story about the power of good becoming victorious over the power of evil. It is the epic and classic plot line that inspires us to rise above.

When you look at this world we live in, power has absolutely been abused, though the lines between "good" and "evil" are not so clear.

Also, generally the characters in each story have to overcome their own "shadows" in order to triumph. The same is true for us.

2. Service to something bigger than ourselves:

In the stories we read, the characters rally together for a cause. Generally, it is to save the world from the forces of evil, which threaten to enslave and destroy all that is good and beautiful. The characters devote themselves completely, with honor and valor, to serve the good of all and bring the world back from the brink of devastation.

This is not so different from the state of our world now. Much is at stake and has already been destroyed. The Earth is on the edge of environmental and political demise, not to mention the publicly unacknowledged groups that want total control and power over everyone else.

But there are a great number of people who are taking a stand, truly dedicating their lives to making this world a better place.

This concept of serving something bigger than yourself adds incredible meaning to your life, allowing you, like the characters in the epic adventures we read, to overcome any challenge and, in doing so, grow stronger and become even more fully who you are.

The Earth is changing, and it is up to each of us to participate in how the future unfolds. We all want to contribute to something bigger and feel that our efforts have made a difference.

This you can do, and this book will help you.

3. Magic and extraordinary abilities

Okay. Magic is always a result of your intention. Always.

Except when magic happens spontaneously, which is rare (we call that *lila* in yoga, which means "Divine play"). If magic is not a result of your own intention, then magic—or anything really—is likely influenced by the intention of another being, seen or unseen.

This has been my experience, and how it has been taught and manifested according to every teacher I have studied with and every book I've read.

Dragons, of course, call to our innate knowing that magic is real and possible for each of us.

It is a scientific fact that we are functioning in this realm, on this level of vibration as human beings, with a fraction of our brain capacity.

There are also millions of accounts of superhuman, psychic, and otherwise unexplainable skills, accomplishments, and occurrences.

These include:

> The ability to see psychic information (Clairvoyance)
>
> The ability to sense psychic information (Clairsentience)
>
> The ability to hear psychic information (Clairaudience)
>
> The ability to be in two places at once
>
> The ability to move objects
>
> The ability to fly
>
> The ability to shape-shift
>
> The ability to telepathically communicate
>
> The ability to co-create and communicate with Nature

And much more…

Magic is very real. Extraordinary things happen all the time.

There is no spoon. (*If you don't get this comment, go watch* The Matrix).
The possibilities are, truly, limitless.

4. Races and beings that are not human

Elves, dwarves, angels, faeries, dragons, spirits, and all manner of other beings, including those from other planets, show up as integral parts of stories in the fantasy realm. Most of the time, the circumstances in the book mean that many or all of these different races have to work together in order to save the world or conquer the villain.

On a surface level, this speaks to the need for all of the different people of the Earth to work together to create a world without war, free from damaging environmental practices, and without the great extremes of poverty and those who have more than they know what to do with.

Each of us is different, but like these different races, we all desire harmony and a life that is in balance with Nature.

Nature herself is teeming with faeries and Nature spirits that many people actually see. All of Nature is sentient. Trees are incredibly powerful, as are crystals, water, mountain spirits, and so on.

Beyond these seemingly obvious correlations, the different races of legends also can be found in the legends of cultures all over the world.

What we know and what science claims to be the history of the world is such a small part of the actual history and timeline of Earth. There were cultures long ago that are now lingering as legend. Think Atlantis and Lemuria, to name only two . . .

The elves could be similar to the "gods" of Egyptian, Mayan, and many other cultures. These are very likely beings from the stars or other dimensions that helped to seed the races of this planet and taught humans all kinds of things, from agriculture to astronomy. Why else would ancient cultures all over the world have incredibly precise astronomical and mathematical building designs, showing an understanding of these sciences that is beyond even what we know today?

If you look into the Great Pyramid, for instance, we don't even have technology today that could replicate it. The enormous structure was not built, as the books tell us, with copper tools and slaves—it's physically impossible. If you delve into the information on just this one monumental building, there is enormous evidence that beings from other planets or stars were behind its construction.

And there are many, many other examples, all over the world, that tell the same tale.

We are not alone.

So that's one possible parallel to the elves, who are generally ancient, with magical powers and understanding beyond human capacity, and who are often "interdimensional" in that they come from or eventually leave the Earth to be in another place that is otherwise unreachable.

There also have been many other ancient races on Earth, traces of which have been left as bones, myths, and artifacts. The dwarves could be an expression of the small Earth dwellers that are at the roots of some indigenous cultures. There are also stories, from many reputable sources, of interdimensional cities and societies living beneath the Earth's surface, under mountains, and even near the Earth's core. Sometimes these inner Earth dwellers are said to be humanoid, and sometimes they are a completely different type of being altogether.

Time and space are enormous.

We understand such a small part of what is, so it only makes sense to expand our idea of what is possible.

The Universe is infinite. We can not be the only life in it.

The races of fantasy gently nudge us in this direction of thinking, so that we can realize that, not only are we not alone, but we need to work together with any other race that desires harmony and balance and peace.

5. Transformation

Don't all the EPIC stories—the ones that capture the imagination and invite you into a different world—occur on the very edge.

One thing turns into another. On subtle and monumental scales. All the time.

Life is a series of transitions, patterns, and flows.

You can't help but notice that the storyline of the apex of an age, where the characters are truly fighting and putting all their effort into saving the world from crumbling, is reflected in what we see around us.

Our personal transformations are constant. We are evolving, expressing ourselves differently. All the time.

Every moment is a choice.

When you begin to think of these elements in the context of how they reflect all around you, it is easier to identify them and realize that your life is far from mundane, so long as you are willing to look for the magic and beauty it contains.

It's simple. And vast in what it signifies.

Concerning Dragons

This book is largely concerned with Dragons and Dragon Riders, and from its pages inquisitive minds and willing spirits can discover much of their character and gain a more comprehensive understanding of their own history.

So let's study Dragons for a bit, shall we?

Dragons, as real beings that exist on some plane of the Universe, are a thrill to connect with and to consult as Guides and friends.

OKAY. FIRST, LET'S ADDRESS THE THRILL PART.

I found this excerpt on a Wiki site online. It does a good job of summing up Dragons as they've been represented in the world of fantasy and literature . . .

> Let's face it: you can't get much more badass than a Dragon. They're huge. They fly. They breathe fire. They have weapons sticking out of nearly every part of their body. They're really, really smart. They're brutal and merciless in battle. They live for thousands of years, they wield magic, and their tough scales make them both pretty and immune to bullets. (Well, it really depends.) As the most well-known and widely overused mythological beast, Dragons have always served as the quintessential boss monster in games, books and myths . . .
>
> . . . Somewhere along the line somebody got the bright idea that maybe these vicious, bloodthirsty beasts don't have to be so evil after all. Maybe underneath all those fangs and claws, they're just gentle, misunderstood creatures who might just be willing to fight on the side of the good guys if you're lucky. In fact, maybe they're just looking for a friend.
>
> And thenceforth, there came the idea of a Dragon Rider, a human (or humanoid) who is so mightily badass he can actually ride on the back of these beasts, often as a steed into battle. The concept exploded and gained ridiculous popularity among fantasy authors, and now can be seen . . . well, just about everywhere in modern fantasy literature.
>
> Dragon Riders are almost always characterized by a bond with the beast they ride which results in a synchronous relationship between the two, a telepathic link, and no possibility that the two could ever be separated from each other without drastic consequences.
>
> *(Source: http://tvtropes.org/pmwiki/pmwiki.php/Main/DragonRider)*

Yep, Dragons are badass.

They're also beautiful, majestic, magical, and incredibly powerful. You can fly on them, and they have personalities so complex that a relationship with them is irrevocably life-changing and soul-expanding.

However you want to picture them, here's the cool part:

DRAGONS ARE REAL.

They are real and a part of our lives, even if we don't yet see them physically in the Third Dimension.

They show up as Guides. They aid us as an unseen influence that works towards empowerment and harmony. They choose to assist us and serve the highest good from their enormous hearts, with ferocious will and enduring love, whether or not we're aware of it.

But who's to say that if we raise our vibrations a bit higher, they won't just magically appear on a tangible level where we could interact with them physically? Or maybe they're hidden in some remote corner of the world, just waiting for us to be ready for them—to BELIEVE in them once more.

Why not? There is so much more to the realm of What Is than what we see and experience in the general idea of a "normal" life.

Dragons, as a symbol, are a delight!

SHAKTI!

Seeing as this is a book about being a Dragon Rider, living fully and guided by the practice of yoga, let's start with Shakti!

Shakti is energy. The supreme creative power that shapes all of life.

She is the Feminine aspect of the One, intertwined with Shiva, who is Divine consciousness.

Shakti breathes your first inhale into you when you are born, and takes your last exhale back into her as you die. Every breath that you receive and give back is the movement of Shakti within.

Energy flows in patterns, can be shifted and directed, and is incredibly intelligent.

When you choose to align with the natural flow of energy, everything in life transpires more smoothly and good things happen. This is a practice, and this Training contains a wealth of ways to work and live in alignment with Nature, completely supported by the Grace of Shakti.

You may have heard of Shakti Kundalini; the coiled inner power within your body that can be awakened, bringing intense insight and limitless possibility.

This awakening happens on its own time, little by little, as you live your practice. It comes in sparks of revelation and moments of incredible beauty. These little illuminations happen all the time.

Kundalini energy is often symbolized as a serpent, and a rising serpent could easily be seen as a Dragon. It is a natural part of you that is simply dormant or subdued most of the time.

It is not something to force, as it can be unsettling if one is unprepared and could unpredictably affect someone who is not ready, just as it would not be wise to push a Dragon around forcibly. Rather, it is by cultivating a relationship of awareness with the energy within that you embrace your inner power and co-participate in a dance of awakening.

As you practice this yoga, you mindfully align with the current of life: the natural flow in the Ocean of Grace.

Being a Dragon Rider is living in the flow of Shakti, one with the current.

I was once told this by a wise man from India:

> *If you unfurl your sails to the winds of Shakti*
> *you will always have enough energy—you can do anything,*
> *for the flow of Shakti carries you.*

Now I say, unfurl your wings!

THE SERPENT

The serpent stands for immense and powerful cosmic movements. This is true of these archetype serpents deep under the Earth, deep under the oceans, on the Earth's surface and in the sky. In fact, it is the very ability of serpents to move between various worlds and different dimensions, as indicated by their hibernation in winter and their life on and in the Earth, which gives them the significance to provide purpose and direction to ways of knowing and being, world-wide. Other physical and transformational qualities of serpents such as the shedding of their skins and regeneration add to the significance of complex, mutable characteristics, and the awe with which they are regarded.

(Source: Nancy C. Maryboy, http://cosmicserpent.org/about-us/the-cosmic-serpent)

Think of a picture of a snake with its tail in its mouth. The image speaks deeply of the cycles of change and transformation.

Dragons and serpents carry much of the same symbolism and powers, for Dragons are the serpents of the sky.

Everyone Knows What A Dragon Looks Like

One of my favorite books when I was a young girl was a children's book called *Everyone Knows What a Dragon Looks Like*, written with a sly wit by Jay Williams and splendidly illustrated by Mercer Mayer.

THE STORY: *EVERYONE KNOWS WHAT A DRAGON LOOKS LIKE*

The main character is a young boy named Han, and his job is to sweep the gate of the city. He lives in a very small hut next to the gate and gets one bowl of rice and one cup of wine every day. He gives each person coming and going a kind word because that is all he has to give.

He lives in a hill village perched between China and the wild. One day a man runs through the gate bringing news of impending doom; the Wild Horsemen of the north are on their way to invade the village.

Han brings the messenger to the Mandarin of the city, and between the Mandarin and his council, they decide the "most practical" answer to the problem is to pray to the Great Cloud Dragon for help.

So the city prays.

And the next day, just before the enemy is in sight, a short, round, old man with a long beard and a staff shows up. In their friendly conversation he tells Han he is a Dragon.

When Han says that the old man doesn't look like a Dragon, the old man asks Han how he's so sure. Has he ever seen one?

And this innocent, humble boy realizes that he hasn't. So he kindly leads the old man up the hill to the palace, where the men in power send him away rudely because they all think they know what a Dragon looks like, and they are all very sure about themselves.

So Han takes the old man to his little hut and offers him his meal for the day, which is all he has to offer for hospitality. For his kindness, the Dragon decides to save the village, even though the men at the top insulted him. He decides it is worth saving the village for this one humble boy who lives his life from a perspective of patience, goodwill, and a pure heart.

The old man goes out and breathes a great wind across the hills where the enemy is galloping in, and the entire army goes flying. The Dragon takes out the whole threat in one breath.

And once his work is done, the small, fat, old man ascends into the sky and transforms into a magnificent Dragon in the clouds. And the whole city, including the men at the top, stand in wonder, gratitude, and respect, for now they all know what a Dragon looks like.

The end of the story is a double-page illustration that exudes peace, with a faint image of a Dragon with its tail in its mouth, forming a circle around a crescent moon.

The Significance

Here we have some of the main threads of the symbolism and powers Dragons (and stories about Dragons) carry:

- ⁓ Transformation of the Self and the World
- ⁓ Integrity of Character
- ⁓ God-like Powers
- ⁓ Rite of Initiation
- ⁓ Overcoming great challenges in remarkable ways
- ⁓ Values of humility, service, kindness, and willingness to see things from a different perspective

And these are just a few examples. As you read, you will identify the significance that is most real and true for you right now. Think of it as a rite of passage as you approach Initiation as a Dragon Rider.

Be mindful and open to realize the significance you see in these words and the story I've just summarized for you. As well as all around you.

Connect with Your Dragon

First, sit beautifully and take three deep breaths. When you feel centered, continue:

See and feel a pure, loving white light surround you and expand within you, from your heart and central core through every cell and extending beyond your skin.

Feel the Earth beneath you, grounding and supportive.

Take another deep breath and notice the change in how you feel.

Now, invite your Dragon, who has already chosen you for who you are in your heart, to introduce itself.

You might feel a shift in energy if you are sensitive, or you might get a message or image that comes to you. However, even if you don't perceive anything, with a clear intention to recognize and know your Dragon, you will be connected on some level.

Take a few breaths to connect to a sense of joyful, powerful love. Your Dragon is a very pure being of great light—that's where its power comes from.

Imagine yourself forming a bond with your Dragon that allows you to communicate, feel, and co-create with it, and also allows you to fly!

Imagine the incredible freedom and joy of flying!

See yourself soaring over the Earth.

Feel the Dragon's scales beneath you, and the rush of wind through your hair (and perhaps some butterflies in your stomach).

What is the landscape you're flying over?

What does your Dragon look like?

What is its name?

What are the qualities of its character?

Might want to write your answers down.

Oh, by the way, you'll want to have a Rider's Journal with you as you go through this Training Manual—the contemplation above is a great first entry.

MORE ON THAT IN YOUR FIRST INITIATION . . .

The First Initiation:
Intention

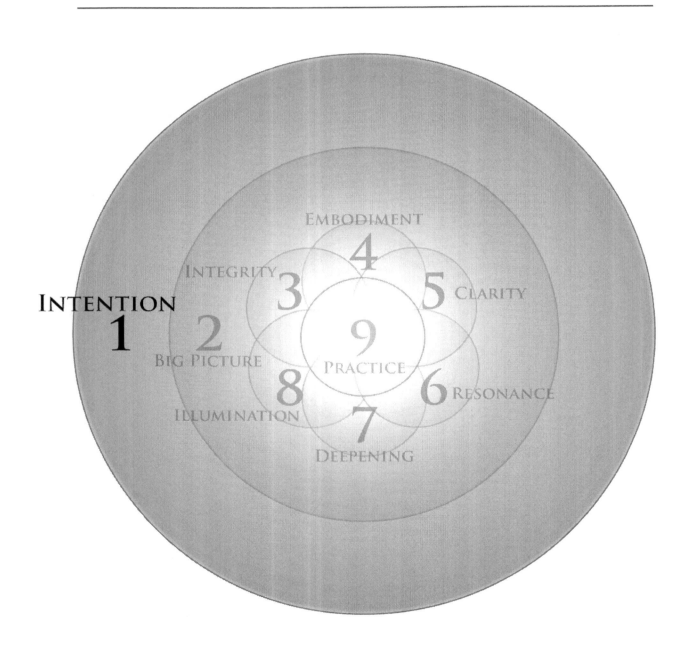

Know Thyself

In order to set out on a journey, it is helpful to first know where you are going. Otherwise you are likely to become lost, confused, and sidetracked unnecessarily.

This Training Manual is divided into sections, and each section is an Initiation.

It is important to complete each section before proceeding to the next Initiation. Otherwise the skills and understanding you need will be incomplete.

That said, it is essential to note that this is a book of *practices*, and you are not expected to perfect any of them before moving on to the next. In fact, if you were to attempt to perfect only one section in this Manual at a time you would do yourself a disservice because they all work together.

You can reference different sections and even play the following game to gain insight. However, it is still of significant importance that you study each section in the order they are presented.

THE SEEMINGLY RANDOM GAME OF INSIGHT

This game is the exception to the rule above.

Yes, you must follow the order of Initiation as you proceed through the sections of this Manual.

However . . .

You may also occasionally play this game to spark your imagination and gain immediate insight, though you may just as easily find riddles as you find clarity and direction.

> *What You Do:*
>
> 1. Think of a question, or don't. You may play this game with specific goals in mind, or you may play for the simple curiosity of playing.
>
> 2. Take a deep breath, and pause in stillness for a moment.
>
> 3. Flip to any page, seemingly at random, and open. You will *know* when to open the book. Your intuition will guide you to the right page.
>
> 4. Read what you find there.
>
> 5. Sit with it. Contemplate. See what comes up and what it means for you.

What You Will Need for this Dragon Rider's Training

There are a few practical tools you will need to begin and get the most out of your practice.

~ A Rider's Journal (or Yoga Diary or whatever you want to call it). Dedicate a notebook to this Adventure of the Self, and use it often to record ideas, experiences, and contemplations that relate to your practice and process.

~ A Yoga Mat. This is your sacred space; home base.

~ A Blanket. You will use the blanket to sit on and also to stay warm. You could even use a cloak if you'd like. I meditate wrapped in my cloak each morning and use it often as a blanket in yoga, though a firmly folded blanket is better support when used underneath you.

~ Yoga blocks and other props (optional). Blocks can be useful tools, especially if your hamstrings are tight. Other helpful props are a strap and a bolster. Instead of a strap you can use a tie, towel, or belt. Instead of a bolster you can use pillows or folded blankets.

Know Your Lineage

Before I go much further, it is important that you know the lineage from which much of this Training originated.

What I present here is a tapestry of wisdom. Each thread that I've woven into this tapestry comes from the many teachers, schools, and practices that inform my own understanding and skills.

I have had many great teachers, and my teachers have had many great teachers. And their teachers have been informed by greatness, which continues through time as the influence of Masters over hundreds of generations.

All of my teachers have influenced my style of teaching, as has all of life around me.

YOGA

I have had many teachers. So many. All of life and every person I have known has been my teacher. I have a brilliant list of people to whom I am grateful in the back of this book.

What has become apparent to me, however, is that you are your own guru. So, as you walk your path, learn from and love many, but never give your power away or defer to someone in a power position. There are different roles when one person is a teacher and one is a student, but equality and integrity are expected from both parties at all times. Giving away power and/or mis-using power creates disharmony. The practice of yoga shows us how to come into harmony, and it's important to cultivate in this every relationship.

My yoga background has ridden many waves. My first class was hot yoga. After that first class I went for a six hour hike to the top of the Chief in Squamish, BC and felt like I was on top of the world. When the teachers at that studio shifted from Bikram into Power Yoga, Yin, and Ashtanga, I tried it all. When I moved to another town I continued to find teachers of a Vinyasa style, and then I found Anusara® yoga. It felt like coming home. I went all-in and committed to six years of incredible personal growth and extensive training.

Anusara yoga has contributed significantly to the innovation and evolution of yoga today, and I am proud to have reached the level of skill necessary to hold a certificate in this method of teaching. Much of what is included in this book is influenced by this school of Hatha yoga. Developed and founded by John Friend, Anusara yoga has flourished and thrived because of the great skill and dedication of many talented teachers. The principles of this system teach optimal alignment and are very effective.

Now I've really stepped into owning my experience with yoga, and teach from the heart using ideas from many sources. It's all about finding your path and dancing into being more fully yourself.

Many people inspire me and have contributed greatly to my own wealth of knowledge of yoga's physical and philosophical practices. Some of the yoga and philosophy teachers who have called to my heart the strongest and taught me the most include Shane Perkins, Douglas Brooks, Jordan Kirk, Cat McCarthy, Denise Benitez, Elizabeth Rainey, Elena Brower, and Rumi . . .

Rather than give you one specific style of yoga in this book, I instead offer you my understanding of yoga in a more general way—which you can then apply to your own practice in the ways that are best for you.

I have also brought in teachings from many other places, a majority of which are presented in the Illumination section. Though these practices don't necessarily come from the tradition of yoga, they integrate beautifully into the vision of oneness that is central to all that yoga teaches.

AKASHIC RECORDS AND INTERDIMENSIONAL INFLUENCE

I learned how to read the Akashic Records from Juliette Looye. Since then, my primary teachers have been those I've been in contact with IN the Records. There are also many light-beings I communicate with on a regular basis through my own inner knowing and intuitive abilities.

These teachers include:
- My Masters, Teachers, and Loved Ones (my Guides)
- Trees and the Plant Kingdom
- The Mineral Kingdom (Crystals)
- The Animal Kingdom (including Dragons!)
- Archangels
- Elementals such as Air, Earth, Fire, and Water
- Deities such as Shiva, Shakti, Lakshmi, Vesta, and Gaia
- Masters such as Christ, Krishna, Mary, Portia, and Quan Yin
- Places of power on the Earth such as sacred sites, the Amazon, oceans, forests, and mountains

Light and Energy Work

I have collected various ways of working with light and energy from many teachers, from shamanic practitioners to Reiki Masters, intuitives and psychic healers. Some of the teachers who stand out in my mind are Scott Marmostein, Michelle Morrison, Antera and Omaran, and Wendy Grono.

The practices I use and teach all come from a strong lineage and are excellent as tools you can apply directly, and ideas you can use as ways to contribute to your own style and preference.

Just as my practice and teachings are uniquely my own, so yours will be.

However, it is very helpful to know the paths and lives and energies that have contributed.

By honoring those who have walked before and those who have been in service of the whole, or the greater good, we remember that we are a part of something bigger.

It helps us remain humble.

The Map Room

Imagine yourself standing in a bright, spacious room. There is a great map on the wall before you and an ornate rug on the floor beneath you.

Sunlight streams in through the windows, illuminating the map. Walk over to it, and take some time to study the journey you are about to undertake.

Though this map is set out in circles rather than mountains, rivers, lakes and oceans, it is an excellent guide on your journey to becoming a Dragon Rider through your practice of yoga.

See yourself standing in this room, before a cryptic treasure of a map.

Know that you are being shown a successful, systematic approach to unlocking secrets and progressing on the path before you.

READY YOURSELF FOR AN ADVENTURE!

The Journey

The First Initiation: **Intention.** *Know Thyself.*

The Second Initiation: **Big Picture.** *Soaring High Above.*

The Third Initiation: **Integrity.** *Shape Your Character.*

The Fourth Initiation: **Embodiment.** *Align, Breathe, Move.*

The Fifth Initiation: **Clarity.** *Cultivate Focus and Contentment.*

The Sixth Initiation: **Resonance.** *The Power of Vibration, Words, and Mantra.*

The Seventh Initiation: **Deepening.** *Weaving Philosophy and Reality Together.*

The Eighth Initiation: **Illumination!** *Working with Light and Energy.*

The Ninth Initiation: **Practice.** *Continuing the Pursuit of Mastery.*

The Map

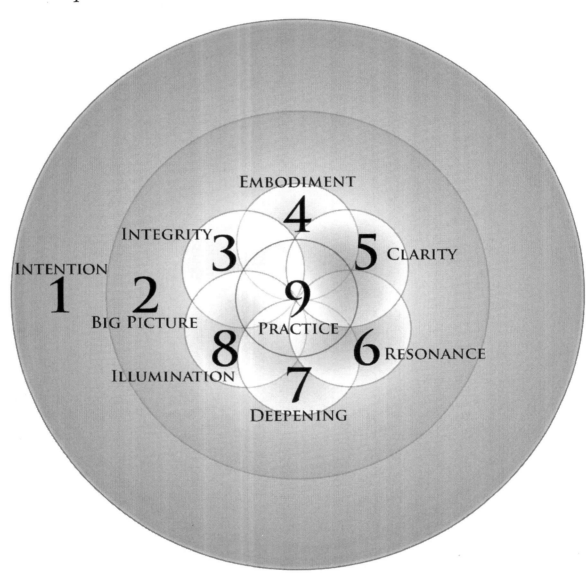

Why Initiations?

You can see that this book is broken into sections called Initiations.

This is because the journey of incorporating all of these different ideas and practices into your life takes time and integration, and it's best to layer things so you can learn more quickly. You will step over an inner threshold as you begin each phase of this Training, coming more fully into balanced power informed by love and wisdom.

Each segment of learning spirals you closer to the inner circle of knowing and ability, where the practice is integrated more and more as a cohesive whole.

As you pass each stage, you progress to the next level of Initiation.

Take your time incorporating each idea and practice, yet remain dedicated to the journey. It is imperative that you continue through every gateway to reach the Sanctuary of the Heart in the center.

When you reach the Ninth Initiation, you will be a Dragon Rider.

You will know what it means to be a Dragon Rider: to live powerfully, with purpose, in the very highest integrity.

The First Initiation, then, is to Set Intention and Know Thyself.

KNOW THYSELF

What is your intention for being here—alive at this time on Earth?

What are your dreams for this journey? What is your mission; your purpose?

What qualities do you want to embody and cultivate?

What experiences do you want to bring more fully into your life and character?

You may not know the answers to these questions right now, but see what ideas come to mind. Your answers may change as time passes and you develop your practice.

Also, keep in mind that part of knowing who you are is developing and nurturing yourself. If you take care of yourself first and remember to stay balanced, you'll find it much easier to take care of others. Many of the practices in this Manual will help.

Character Contemplation

Who do you want to be?

Sometimes the answer to this is not immediately forthcoming. So a good question to ask yourself in this case is *Who Do I Admire?*

What are the traits you admire in others—people you know or don't, living or not, in reality or in a book, movie or dream?

Listing some of their most admirable traits and abilities will give you a good idea of what you can cultivate within yourself.

Here is a list I came up with years ago. You may use what inspires you:

- ~ Honorable
- ~ Joyful
- ~ Beautiful
- ~ Magical
- ~ Loving
- ~ Kind
- ~ Thoughtful
- ~ Strong yet soft
- ~ Courageous
- ~ Intelligent
- ~ Patient
- ~ Full of acceptance
- ~ Powerful
- ~ Wise
- ~ Wealthy
- ~ Eagle-eyed
- ~ Total clarity in focus and thought
- ~ A great healer
- ~ Celebrated singer-songwriter
- ~ Able to play many instruments
- ~ Able to speak many languages (especially the powerful essence—Sanskrit)
- ~ Able to meditate deeply and easily
- ~ Able to see, move, feel, hear, and work with energy
- ~ Able to walk across worlds/dimensions freely, safely, easily
- ~ Always in the flow of Grace
- ~ An honored, humble, masterful teacher

When you identify the qualities and virtues you wish to embody, you can weave them into your intention.

It is interesting, to me, when I look back on these types of contemplations in my journal, to find that I now embody all of them to a certain extent, even if I have yet to bring every one to complete Mastery.

Your Dragon

Remember in the last section, in the "Connect with Your Dragon" exercise, how you envisioned exactly what your Dragon would be like and what it would feel like to have a relationship with a Dragon?

Well, go back and answer those questions if you haven't already, and write them down in your Rider's Journal.

They will help you visualize and more skillfully venture forward as a Dragon Rider.

Your Name

Your name says much about you. Yes, you have a name that you were given at birth, however I believe that on some level you influenced the choice of that name.

But even beyond your birth name, you have other names, and you may also take a name of your choosing. Again, you do not have to decide now, but it may be fun to jot down some ideas that please you.

Remember to write the date each time you make an entry in your Rider's Journal. As your name and intention may change, knowing when you wrote the entry helps you look back and understand yourself more fully, as well as track your progress along your journey.

If you go back to the Invitation in the first section of this book, you can re-read the segment titled Who Am I? This gives you examples of my own names, and ideas that you can use to discover more fully what your name and your purpose means to you.

Intention

Your focus shapes your world. Your intent shapes your focus.

When you are clear about your purpose, what you want to create, and where you want to go, you empower yourself.

By setting your intention, aligning with it, and bringing it into the world through word and action, life flows.

And the Universe conspires to manifest the life you choose.

Of course, your Dragon helps . . .

Integrating the First Initiation

In order to leave The Map Room and move on to the next step, you must have some idea of where you are going.

You need to set an intention so you can venture onward.

Write your intention down and speak it out loud.

You may already even know what it is.

The questions and examples below offer ideas should you want them.

Set Your Intention

What is your intention for being here—alive at this time on Earth?

What are your dreams for this journey? What is your mission; your purpose?

What qualities do you want to embody and cultivate?

What experiences do you want to bring more fully into your life and character?

It can be as simple as:

> *I choose light, love, joy and peace.*
> *I choose happiness and health, beauty and wealth.*

It can be as specific as:

> *I am strong, wise, and skillful, living my life fully with a playful spirit and an open heart. I am pure and protected, powerful and humble. I intend to study and practice with my whole self, so that I may know myself as whole and complete.*

It can be as long as the following poem, which was my intention on the autumnal equinox of 2010, at the full moon, written just after sunrise.

I choose health and wealth
    love and light
    joy and laughter
    peace and beauty

I choose to be a blessing
    to myself
    to this planet
    to all the Divine children
        who play upon it

I choose to live in the one
    Truth and magic
    of the Here and Now

I am a sage
    I am a child of God
        I am that I am

I welcome the highest goodness
    and Grace
    into my life
        in abundance

I dance this grand game in gratitude
    In harmony with All That Is

Om Namah Shivaya
    Om Shri Lakshmi Namaha
        Om Shri Shakti Namaha Ma Ma Ma
            Om*Amen*

However you phrase it, have some clear idea of where you want to go and what you want to create as you take this journey.

Powerful words to begin your phrasing include:

- ~ I am . . .
- ~ I intend . . .
- ~ I choose . . .
- ~ May I . . .

Be sure to write down your intention in your Rider's Journal. To make it even more powerful, speak it out loud.

Journal as often as you want. Record your experiences, feelings, and observations as you begin and continue your yoga practice.

By writing things down, you get a bigger-picture understanding of who you are, what life is, and how your relationship with yourself and everything around you is ever-evolving.

The more you know who you are, the more authenticity you bring to living your purpose, and the more you can contribute your own talents and find joy in everything you do.

Notice how your intention grows and changes as you yourself grow and change with the practices you learn here.

The Second Initiation:
Big Picture

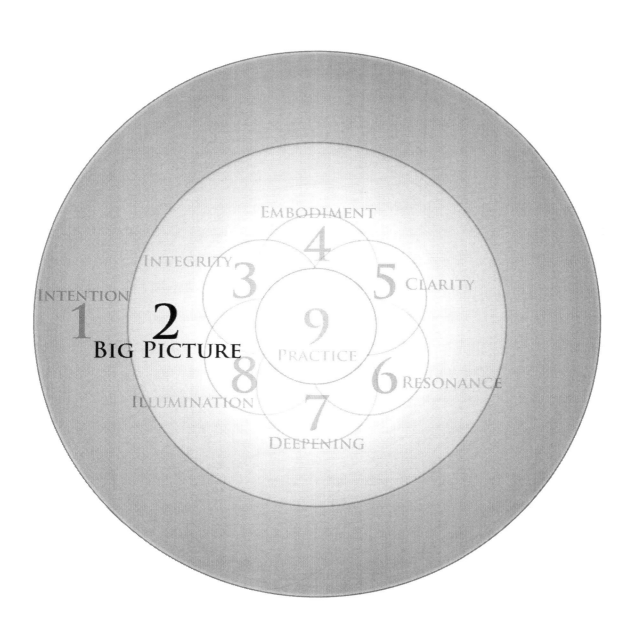

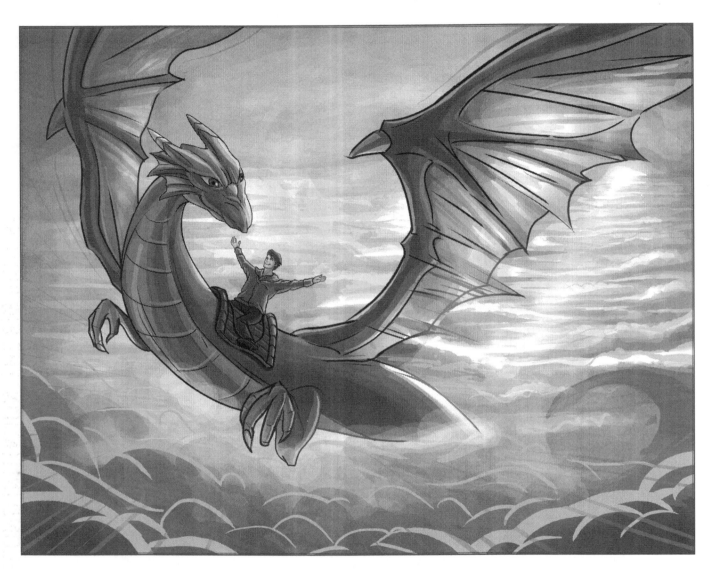

Out beyond ideas of wrongdoing and rightdoing, there is a field. I'll meet you there.

—Rumi

Soaring High Above

Okay. So the idea of being able to do magic, riding and telepathically linked to a Dragon, is pretty cool.

It brings two entirely different beings together to work as one. It allows a completely different perspective and ability to see a bigger picture of life on many levels.

The weaving and working together of one being and another creates a bond that intrigues in its ability to symbolize many things at once, as does the concept and experience of flying.

CONSIDER THE IDEA OF BEING A DRAGON RIDER FROM THESE THREE PERSPECTIVES:

1. With a big picture view (everything is one)
2. On an embodied level (envisioning yourself as a Dragon Rider)
3. As an Individual with many layers (an interdimensional being)

And as your perspective changes, even though you are still considering the same one concept of Dragon and Rider, you will notice many things. It's a very good idea to jot some of these things down. In your Rider's Journal, write out the elements that speak most strongly to your heart and your sense of who you are, as well as who you want to be.

What a Dragon Rider sees and experiences—the Big Picture:

- Oneness, union, interconnectedness
- Connected to a greater energy
- Co-creating with the Divine
- Attuned to Nature, supported by Grace
- Freedom, liberation, beauty
- Joy, happiness, laughter, play
- Gratitude, trust, acceptance
- Expansive power
- Fullness, vastness, wholeness
- Bird's-eye view; Dragon's-eye view
- Humility, equanimity
- Releasing limiting ideas
- Clarity, focus, perspective
- Ability to be present, living in the now
- Feeling grounded and light
- Open awareness, listening

~ Devotion, expressing gratitude for life

~ Centeredness, contentment, creativity

~ Expanded possibilities

~ Authenticity, calling forth your truth

Using Yoga to See the Big Picture

The last exercise gets you thinking big picture. This is an essential ability to cultivate in order to live life skillfully and fully.

The first thing you do in yoga is pause, feel, and be sensitive. Feel your breath move.

By doing so, you connect to a bigger energy—that which you already know as true in your heart—the sentient, pulsating force of life.

Yoga means "union," which is particularly fitting when you consider it from the concept of being a Dragon Rider, shattering limiting beliefs that make you think you are separate and alone. You're not.

However, the oneness that is the grand purpose of yoga is a union so complete that it goes far beyond the idea of Dragon and Rider . . .

Unless you look at it like this:

The Dragon symbolizes the Divine; the conscious, creative energy that expresses itself by manifesting infinitely as you, as everything you know and see, and all else as well.

Being a Dragon Rider is complete union between the Individual and the Universal.
It is realizing that you are an expression of the Divine, and conducting yourself as such.

This Universal power and sentience is the One that has become the many. It is everything in the Universe and also holds the Universe within itself.

It has been called many names, and you must name it what is best for you. I interchange Nature, Universe, Divine, God, Grace, Spirit, Energy, and many more.

The name matters and also does not, for what we are talking about here is beyond description and normal comprehension.

That's why this works so well:

By engaging your imagination as a Dragon Rider, you fly above the barrier of thought patterns that muddy the mind and confuse the thoughts on such a vast and significant concept.

When you seek union with this bigger energy—through your breath, through your awareness, through the practice of yoga and of being human—Spirit comes to you. Nature embraces you with her infinite arms. The sparks of magic are found in every element of life. You bond with your Dragon, bringing indescribable delight!

Sit beautifully for a few moments in stillness. Read this a few times and FEEL it within you.

Contemplation

Breathe and let yourself be breathed into your fullness.

Be complete in the magic of the moment, and make that magic your new realm, your new way.

Let the wind and the breath of God clear away the veil of limiting beliefs to uncover who you really are!

You ARE the Divine.

See yourself as such. Perceive all things from this perspective.

Open to Nature and align with her flow.

It is time for you to claim your full power.

You are ready. You are loved. You are supported. You are guided.

Now is the time to BE.

Entering the Philosophy of the Big Picture

There are ways to learn how to flow with the waves of life so that you can go gracefully along for the ride, skillfully living with the changes and challenges that come.

This is what the philosophical approach of yoga is about. When you learn to align with the current of Nature, you tap into the awakening and freedom that people have been seeking throughout the ages and legends.

Let's simplify the philosophy that really allows you to bring more ease and enjoyment into your life, shall we?

FIRST THINGS FIRST. GO BIG PICTURE.

Imagine you're soaring high above and can see the world beneath you. Seeing from this Dragon's-eye view invites you to open to the bigger energy that pulses and dances as everything. This feeling of being connected to something bigger reminds you that you're not alone, that everything is interconnected, and you can actually align with this bigger energy in a way that is life-enhancing and empowering.

This perspective brings a sense of equanimity and humility. It allows you to step back and collect yourself so you can choose to think, speak, and behave in ways that support a life of goodness and integrity.

When you remember to be sensitive and spacious—to tune in to the pulsing Spirit of life, then you can make more skillful choices and experience more delight.

First, Be Open

What does it mean to be open to life?

It means that you're open to see and consider all possibilities. That you first broaden your perspective and remember that there is always a gift or blessing being offered in every moment, no matter how painful or messy or strange the situation might be.

Then, once you've been receptive to what is possible, you can define what parts of life you want to stay open to, and those you don't. First you open, then you set clear and healthy boundaries by making your own choices about what is best for you.

When you recognize that you have this choice to pause and reconnect with something bigger than your Individual idea of yourself, things change. You start to make choices that are life-affirming, bigger-picture decisions.

You take the blinders off and see the world in a different light.

This doesn't mean you're always happy and ignore the pain of your own life or the suffering of the world. Instead, you acknowledge what is going on, and endeavor to RESPOND rather than REACT.

And here's the real skill that you can learn or may already be practicing: learning to discern between response and reaction.

When you REACT to what happens, it's more like a reflex, and chances are the habitual negativity that is so much a part of mass media and social conditioning will influence that reaction. When you RESPOND to what is, it is a conscious choice.

Practicing yoga, on and off the mat, keeps you coming back to this idea of opening up to the Universal before getting into the necessary identification of the Individual elements of life.

You choose to align with the auspicious, conscious energy that pulsates within you and all around you. You practice widening your perspective so you can recognize the inherent goodness in others and yourself.

Living from a Big Picture Perspective: Looking for the Beauty

Open to feel the bigger energy.

Feel your breath.

Connect consciously through your intention of aligning with the flow of life.

Expand your awareness and train yourself to look for what is good and beautiful in this moment and every moment.

Then CHOOSE that which is most life-affirming—that which will bring the greatest amount of delight in the highest sense of the word.

Open. Align. Embrace. (Repeat.)

See the gift in each moment, be open to receive it, and then act upon it in the way that holds the most integrity and is aligned with your own truth.

Be Here Now

Many years ago, I discovered a magical book on my parents' shelf.

I was standing there, gazing up at the top-right corner, and I saw this purple book. I pulled it out. There was a mandala of sorts on its cover, with a very elaborate star, a chair, and the words *Be Here Now* circling around. I became enthralled with this copy of *Be Here Now* by Ram Dass ($3.33, published 1971, Year of the Earth Monkey, seven years before I was born).

My dad laughed good-naturedly at my discovery and presented it to me to keep. Most of the book is illustrated and dancing with contemplations and wisdom. I do believe I took that book to a month-long yoga teacher-training, where I fell asleep each night listening to the sound of the ocean and awakened at dawn each day. The book didn't actually get a whole lot of use while I was there, but when I did open it, I got a lot out of the simple wisdom I read.

One of my favorite quotes from it is:

> *When you know how to listen*
> *Everybody is the Guru.*

Be. Here. Now.

The magic is in the moment. Presence is truly All That Is.

One of the things I learned from the ocean that month was how to flow. How to be present. How to allow the song of my heart to come through.

In the words of my beloved teacher and heart brother, Shane Perkins:

> *Show Up. Let Go.*

> *Show Up. Let Go.*

> *Show Up. Let Go.*

When you are in the moment, worries and overwhelm dissolve. Don't grasp at what has come before. Don't try to pull at what has not yet come to be.

Be here. Now.

And simply do your best in every moment. It always will be perfect.

About the Akashic Records

Imagine a Library in Heaven.

It holds all information. No document has ever been lost or burned. No idea forgotten.

Akasha is the Sanskrit word for space, sky, ether, heaven.

The Akashic Records are the information that has been collected from every impression on the landscape of space-time and beyond. Accessing the Akashic Records is a way to communicate with interdimensional beings and Guides to receive information that can inform your life and understanding.

When I "go into the Records," I basically meditate, illuminate my energy field, focus my intention, and connect by way of a specific phrase or collection of phrases. I have learned to attune to the Records through a state of receptivity that allows me to talk with Guides and Masters, Angels and Nature.

Much of the information in the latter part of this book came from the Akashic Records, communicated from higher dimensions. These are tremendous teachings, given with great love and in service of bringing more light to this experience of being human.

Reading the Akashic Records is something that can be learned, something that can be taught. I can even hook you up with my teacher, Juliette Looye. Her information is in the appendices at the end of this book.

A Message from the Akashic Records

Remember to appreciate what you have right now. Move out of "should" and "shouldn't," and into wonder and gratitude. What does the wind sing to you as it blows? What do delays leave time for you to do or see? What opportunities arise in the perceived "un-ideal" circumstances?

And how can you more fully enjoy every single moment? For this is why you are here. This is what the game is about. Not the next place and the next thing, but the NOW. Love to be in it.

Gather all of your talents together and move as one through time and space as a whole being. Then you won't feel scattered and tired. You will advance on your path much more quickly and smoothly. Your growth, your moving forward, comes from the perfection of being here now.

One of the most important things is to be open to what is before you. If your focus is narrow and you're stuck in yourself like a turtle in its shell, you can't see the opportunities that are there.

Even in the darkest hour there is a gift waiting to be recognized.

So the philosophy of this yoga we are exploring teaches you to look for the good and to find the beauty in everything.

Because when you can identify the good in any situation, you can then choose it. That doesn't mean you ignore everything else or pretend that a challenge isn't there, but you can rise above difficulties so much more easily when you align with what is good and right for you.

This one concept is enough to make a big difference in life.

As a Dragon Rider, to shape your character in a way that enhances and enriches your life and life all around you, look for the beauty. Let your perspective be spacious and present, moment-by-moment.

Reading the Akashic Records is not a traditional aspect of yoga or a part of Anusara yoga. It is, however, a very helpful tool to understand who you are and the complexity of life. It can be an excellent complement to your yoga practice, and enhance your ability to stay open to the Big Picture.

Raising Your Vibration

All of the tools you receive in this Training Manual for Dragon Riders—everything you learn on this path of yoga (union)—helps you raise your vibration.

For example, as you resonate at a higher level, you increase power in balance with love and wisdom.

Hatred is a very low frequency. Fear and anger are more low-vibration frequencies.

Love, joy, and peace, are very high frequencies.

The more you align yourself with a perspective and an experience based in these pure expressions of being, the higher your vibration becomes.

When you open to connect with the Source of who you are; when you open who you are as an Individual to the Universal self, you move into a vibration of love and goodness.

Insight naturally comes along the way. And the more you do this—the more you live in a way that brings Divine connection, love, and peace—the higher you raise your vibration.

When your vibration is at a very high level, you can fly!

How to Shift Your Perspective to See Beauty

Most people are conditioned to look for what is wrong in the world. They look for what is different or difficult. They tend to judge first, observe later.

Since what you focus on is what you experience, this is a twisted perspective to teach as a society. It does not lead people towards creating a Golden Age, or even a Happy Life. Of course, you can choose a different way.

Training yourself to see beauty in each moment and thing, even if there is also ugliness and difficulty, is crucial to accepting and realizing that everything you see and experience is an expression of Divine energy.

Looking for beauty is not ignoring the reality of things, because you also want to see clearly and observe things as they are. However, what you do by focusing on beauty is bring more of that goodness into your world.

You create a habit of finding what is life-enhancing, and by focusing on that you choose to support it with your energy and actions.

If you do not look for the beauty in yourself and in the world around you, you will continue to consider yourself as separate.

Focusing on difference and identifying what is "wrong" creates an instinctual reaction to want to pull away in order to protect yourself. It puts up walls and barriers, preventing you from noticing that there are actually similarities, opportunities for compassion, and even beauty to be found. It blocks the truth that all things are interconnected. And it keeps you from accepting and healing parts of yourself that are wounded.

Why would you want to nurture a connection between yourself and the world around you if you don't see beauty and goodness there? You wouldn't.

So, in order to foster an environment within you that acknowledges and accepts that all things are interconnected, you need to be able to see goodness and beauty wherever you look. Sometimes it's challenging, but it is there.

This is how I turned my judgmental mind around. It is also your ongoing homework assignment until it becomes habitual.

THE GAME OF SEEING BEAUTY

Play a game with your perspective.

The object of the game is to train yourself to habitually look first for the good and beauty in any moment, no matter what is before you. You will also see the other elements that are there, but learn to first and foremost see the gift.

As you go through life, identify something good in everything and everyone you see. When you look at yourself in the mirror, or watch your thoughts, what do you see that is wonderful?

When you see someone else, what about them is beautiful?

When you look around you, what in your environment is an artistic expression of life?

When you look at each situation, what opportunity is offered?

Example: As an elderly woman walks slowly in front of you up the street, rather than thinking "This wrinkly old turtle is in my way!" and impatiently looking for a way to get around her, acknowledge the fact that she is out walking around, getting fresh air, and moving her body. Wonderful! Then go ahead and pass her, but as you do so, your awareness of the good she is doing acts as a silent blessing, rather than the frustration and negativity you would have sent her if you were coming from a perspective of judgment.

This example shows how this game of looking for the beauty not only changes your own perspective and experience in life for the better, it also ripples out to shift the energy *around you* in a positive way.

Integrating the Second Initiation

In order to complete this level of your Training, it is important that you can do three things:

1. You understand the concept of going Big Picture—connecting with a bigger energy—and you are willing to continually practice opening to an awareness of the Universal sense of self.
2. You can appreciate the importance and significance of being present in the moment, because "Here and Now" is where life is happening.
3. You are able to identify the beauty around you and endeavor to first look for the good in yourself and all others, and in the world around you.

Assess where you are on these three points.

If you have contemplated these views and habitually practice applying them in your daily life to the best of your ability, then you are well on your way to becoming a gifted Dragon Rider!

Now, the journey continues . . . layering the next part of your Training upon the foundation of the Big Picture.

The Third Initiation:
Integrity

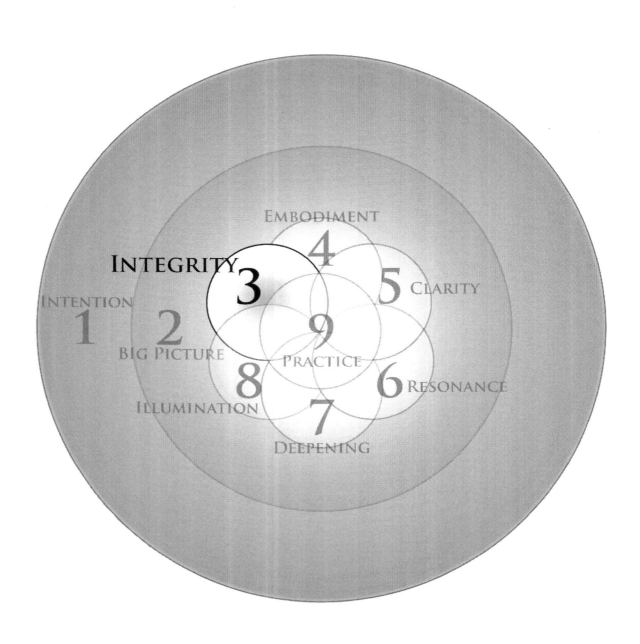

Shape Your Character

Bring your full awareness and attention here and now, for this is the foundation upon which all else is built.

This Initiation, this work that you are about to begin, is potent and life-changing. It will profoundly deepen your ability to act honorably and authentically as a Dragon Rider.

Who do you want to be?

How can you take who you are and become even more of who you want to be?

What are the things that stand in your way?

What attributes of yourself need to be cultivated and empowered? What elements need to be transmuted, or dissolved and dissipated, so that they no longer interfere with your happiness and progress?

This stage of your journey isn't just about asking these questions and pondering their meaning. It's about taking action and making real changes.

You are about to shape your character and become more fully who you have chosen to be.

Are you ready?

You Are Worthy

First things first: it is important to realize that you are beginning from a good place.

Yes, you have habits and traits that need to be shed or shaped in order to polish the gemstone of the heart and free you to experience the fullness of your purpose and power.

However . . .

If you begin from a place of frustration you will only get in your own way.

Instead—and this can sometimes be challenging—you need to know that you are already perfect, in your human imperfections, and that from this place of perfection you can open to unlimited possibility.

The essence of who you are is goodness, light, and love. Even if it doesn't always feel that way.

Self-Acceptance

Unconditional self-acceptance is at the core of a peaceful mind.

This wisdom comes with a story.

Long years ago I was wandering through a forest, singing. The trees were tall and a mighty river flowed near, cold from the snowmelt of the surrounding mountains. The river was so cold that to bathe in it, I had to jump in and out several times and bathe in stages.

I was in that particular forest at that particular time for a festival of sorts. It was a gathering of tribes, a party with multiple stages for music, a village of tents and campers that lasted for a few days and then disappeared. At night there were sparkling lights and the music rang through the valley, echoing off the mountains.

There I danced, witnessed the creation of an elaborate crystal grid, connected with my tribe, explored islands within the river, created a stone labyrinth, and ventured on foot to a nearby clearing where another party was taking place. Just as I arrived fireworks exploded into the night.

On the last day, as I was wandering through the trees sharing my song with them, just enjoying the company of the forest, a faerie came and gave me a small piece of paper. On it was written the eleven words you see here:

Unconditional self-acceptance is at the core of a peaceful mind.

This wisdom, these eleven words marked a turning point in my life because I realized that I did NOT accept myself for who I was. I was judgmental, impatient, and often disappointed in myself. I even, on occasion, dug deep pits of despair and sat in them, using harsh words towards myself and turning my anger inward.

Self-sabotage is not helpful, not useful, and not an honorable way to contribute to uplifting the world. I know this because I have tried it on for size and have been caught in the habitual pattern of it.

This is actually a pretty common experience for many people. And the difference between living in that state of not accepting themselves, compared to shifting their perspective to one of self-acceptance, is the difference between being imprisoned in the dark, compared to watching the sky lighten with the promise of dawn and a radiant sunrise.

I RECEIVED THE FOLLOWING MESSAGE FROM THE AKASHIC RECORDS:

First of all, you already ARE that which you want to be. You just don't experience it fully yet at this stage of the game. You have done and are doing very well. Know that.

Judgment stands in your way. Impatience and expectations set you up for disappointment as well. These are the main roots of anger and clouded vision.

Flying with childlike fun-loving laughter is a wonderful vehicle to take you where you want to go. Wonder, joy; the outlook of curious gratitude for whatever comes, is the way out of the above traps. Stay in and with the love you know is at your essence, and you become and embody it.

Know, without doubt, that you are light, protected by light, surrounded by light, and that only love and light are possible. Believe this as fully as you intellectually know it. Practice it always. You have begun. You are doing well. Keep it up.

When you accept yourself, exactly as you are in each moment, imperfectly perfect, the unlimited possibilities open up to you. You have gotten out of your own way and can choose to make any changes or enhancements in your character and in life that you desire.

You already ARE that which you want to be, in that there is nothing separate from you and everything exists within you. So really, this idea of shaping your character is a practice of choosing what existing parts of yourself and the boundless energy of the Universe you want to embody and express.

The guiding principles of yoga help you do just that, and in a way that becomes habitual, instinctual, and transformational.

The Yamas and Niyamas of Yoga

The yamas and niyamas are, in a nutshell, the ethical foundation of yoga.

They are principles that invite you to raise your level of integrity in a way that enhances, enriches, and empowers your relationship with yourself and the world.

There's something you should know about me.

I've never been a big fan of rules.

Growing up I pretty much rebelled against anyone telling me what to do if I didn't want to do it. That didn't make me a particularly respectful student or daughter sometimes, but that's how I was.

Over time I have learned respect, and now I see that most of my struggles came from a lack of respect for myself and the world around me. I can now interpret or break the rules with tact and finesse . . . at least most of the time.

I'm simply not of a mind to accept arbitrary rules and laws that do not belong to the laws of Nature. I understand why we have them in our societies, but if everyone simply lived lives of integrity and allowed themselves to be guided by ancient wisdom, such as the yamas and niyamas, we could effectively govern ourselves in many ways.

When I first started studying yoga, I found many teachers and books that offered information from a Classical viewpoint, mainly influenced by the great *Yoga Sutras of Patanjali.*

Let me help you understand the differences in approach between Classical philosophy and Tantra, since we'll look at the yamas and niyamas from this point of view.

Basically, Classical Yoga seeks the freedom of enlightenment by practicing yoga to overcome the distractions of the mind and body.

Though much of yoga has evolved from this perspective, it didn't quite jibe with my inner rebel because it felt like parts of me (my body and mind) were problems—less Divine or pure than my spirit.

That just didn't feel quite right, so I took what made sense to me and put the rest on hold.

Then came my first taste of the unifying philosophy of Tantra, and my world, literally, changed overnight.

WHY?

Because Tantra as a philosophy is so beautifully woven, and functions on the principle of taking what works for you and leaving the rest. It is based on a sense of oneness that I already understood as my inner knowing. It absolutely, completely, and delightfully resonated with me. It fit exactly with the things I had already discerned for myself as true: what I already believed in my heart.

There wasn't anything to rebel against because this approach welcomed me as the unique, somewhat strange and radically creative person that I am.

Tantric philosophy essentially describes the entire Universe (including you and me) as an infinite creative expression of the conscious, blissful, essentially good, perfectly and completely free, pulsating energy that is All That Is.

Tantra teaches that ALL of who you are is Divine.

Even those parts of you that can be distracting, fearful, or frustrating.

Why? Because there is nothing other than the Divine. So even those shadows that we deal with as human beings are, at their very essence, rooted in goodness because they help us evolve and develop more fully into who we are.

This makes transformation SO much easier because you can say, "Well, even though I have to work on aligning my body with what I consider ideal, and get my mind to somehow quiet and focus, and even though I make mistakes, I'm still okay!"

Now, to be clear, Classical and Tantric practitioners are all aiming for the same goal, which is to be in full awareness of the oneness of existence, which brings all kinds of good things like deep peace and ecstatic bliss. It's just that the constructs of belief and perspectives they use as they go about it are quite different.

The yamas and niyamas are the guiding ethical principles of yoga. These Empowering Principles of Integrity are elements of character that you naturally align with as you live in high integrity. (And, yes, I came up with the idea of calling them "Empowering Principles of Integrity." Because that's what they are.)

The yamas are the virtues you cultivate as you relate to the world around you. The niyamas are the virtues you cultivate in yourself as an Individual.

They are the natural virtues of a life lived in harmony, from the heart.

So, from the perspective of oneness and goodness, here are the yamas and niyamas:

The Empowering Principles of Integrity
THE YAMAS

Ahimsa (loving kindness)

Satya (truthfulness)

Asteya (non-stealing)

Brahmacharya (unconditional love and highest integrity)

Aparigraha (living simply)

THE NIYAMAS

Saucha (purity)

Santosha (deep contentment)

Tapas (discipline serving delight)

Svadhyaya (deep study of the self and yoga)

Ishvara-pranidhana (deep devotion and joyful surrender)

A NOTE ON SANSKRIT AND STUDYING THE SUTRAS

In each section, I've included the Sanskrit words and interpretations for the yamas and niyamas as they appear in *The Yoga Sutras of Patanjali*, an ancient text studied by all serious students of yoga.

Sanskrit holds incredible power. As you study the Sanskrit sutras, say each sutra out loud a few times and notice how the resonance feels.

Sometimes the sutras are written as one long word with all the individual words running together. To make it easier for you to speak and study these sutras, I have put hyphens between words so you can see them more clearly.

The three main sources I have studied for this are *Light on the Yoga Sutras of Patanjali* by B.K.S. Iyengar, *The Heart of Yoga* by T.K.V. Desikachar, and my studies and many trainings with John Friend. I encourage you to explore other perspectives in addition to what you find here.

Be unafraid. Sanskrit is more or less pronounced the way it is written, and it is not of dire consequence to get it exactly right as you are learning. There are many ways to write and translate Sanskrit, and I am not the authority on this so I have simply presented things as they make sense to me. You can refine as your practice unfolds. Do your best and delight in this adventure of sacred, ancient wisdom as it applies directly to your life and purpose.

The Yamas and Niyamas

Ahimsa: Loving Kindness

Though *ahimsa* is generally translated as "non-harming" or "non-violence," the scope of what it can offer you is vast and potent.

Why? Because what ahimsa is really doing is inviting you to live from the perspective and experience of loving kindness, compassion, and the ability to flow with the current and goodness of Nature.

Not being violent or harmful towards others is common sense; obvious to most of us. But it's the more subtle areas that take practice and can bring such personal transformation.

It's where the lines blur that you really need the inner guidance of ahimsa.

How can you have an attitude of loving kindness towards people who have done great harm to the world or to you personally? How do you know what to choose when things aren't so clear?

This is a very high practice, and the endeavor is self-healing while it also creates an influence of healing and harmony on a vibratory level that impacts the world.

Ahimsa is finding the way of love on the path that is most aligned with your heart.

When you're in a situation that's a bit sticky to figure out, ask your heart these questions:

What is the choice that honors the essential goodness of life? What flows with Nature? What feels right?

And then, as you make your choice, remember that how you go about it also makes a difference.

For example, I recently began integrating meat into my diet after many years of eating vegetarian and sometimes raw-vegan diets. I found that my health and energy weren't where I wanted them to be, and I was craving meat for two months before I finally acted on that inner guidance. It was a tough choice.

Yes, eating meat involves killing animals, which is definitely violent and harmful. This is one reason why yoga generally instructs a vegetarian diet. And there are all kinds of environmental considerations about how the animals are raised. But by choosing local, free range, hormone- and nitrate-free meat, I can minimize the harm done because I'm at least supporting humane animal husbandry rather than factory farming. And by not eating more than I need—I still eat mostly vegetarian—I reduce my footprint and the amount I contribute to the suffering of animals.

By eating with deep respect and gratitude, and by blessing my food as well as the other animals that are destined for the same fate, I can actually add love into the cycle.

> *May all animals be blessed. May they live joyful lives of peace and comfort.*
> *May they feel my gratitude. May they enjoy the sun, pure water, the peace of Earth, and*
> *the beauty of life.*

This kind of intention not only raises the vibration of my meal, it also ripples out on some subtle level to influence the quality of life of the animals who are raised for meat or fish who are caught wild in the oceans, as well as those who are not. However long they are alive, may they enjoy the experience. May it be good for them.

Gandhi, Metta, and Embodying Ahimsa

Buddhism works with loving kindness as Metta, which is a beautiful practice of unconditional loving kindness, compassion, and goodwill.

You can embody the deep loving kindness of a bodhisattva and the transformational influence of peace that we so appreciate from Gandhi's life. When you need help in your practice of being human and living ahimsa, simply picture Gandhi, Buddha, or anyone you identify with who has mastered loving kindness.

By focusing on this inner image of ahimsa as perfected by a great Master, you will start to resonate with that whole and evolved expression of it, and your own energy will shift.

As you become more and more Masterful at embodying and radiating loving kindness, you do the world a great service and increase the presence and power of goodness and Grace. This is one of the roles a Dragon Rider willingly serves as an offering to the interconnectedness of all of life.

Sutra 2.35: ahimsa-pratisthayam tat sannidhau vaira-tyagah

Ahimsa	non-violence
Pratisthayam	standing firmly, well established (pra=on + stha=stand)
Tat	his/her
Sannidhau	presence, vicinity
Vaira	animosity, hostility
Tyagah	forsaking, abandoning, deserting

This sutra states that when you have firmly established non-violence in thought, speech and action, your own aggression dissolves and others abandon hostility in your presence.

When your practice of ahimsa becomes your Nature—when it Guides your words, your thoughts, and your actions toward yourself and others—you become a power of peace. You create a vibration of life-enhancing harmony that affects the world around you.

May all beings be happy.

May all beings be free from suffering.

May all beings live lives of joy, love, and peace.

Satya: Living Your Truth

Satya, or "truthfulness," invites you to be genuine—authentic to your inner Nature with integrity and complete honesty. This is the second of the yamas.

A large part of satya is being truthful with yourself. When you are authentically you, it is naturally beautiful; it feels good.

It might not be comfortable at first to genuinely express who you are because most of us have been brought up conditioned to "fit in" and go with some outside definition of normal . . . whatever that is.

But when you are around people who are completely living their truth with integrity, knowing who they are, their confidence is palpable, their inner beauty radiant, and the feeling of being with them often evokes delight.

When you live your truth, you stop fighting the flow of life because you are honoring your true Nature as a unique expression of Divine life.

On the other hand, pretending to be who you are *not* can be rather difficult and can bring suffering to you and those around you.

It's one thing to try on a costume and play with a role to see what parts of it speak to you and fit your needs, but to deny yourself, to hide your genuine self . . . It's like taking a masterpiece of art—a Picasso, say—and shrouding it in a dusty corner of a broom closet.

It does not serve the glory of this incredibly, magnificently diverse experience we call life to be anyone but who you are.

GROWING PAINS AND SATYA AS SELF-HONESTY

Part of being truthful with yourself is honestly acknowledging the places you need to grow. This is simply the process of being human, as we all have things to work on.

It isn't always easy, but if you are truthful with yourself (satya), and you practice loving kindness (ahimsa) supported by the many tools of yoga, the growing evolution of who you are will bring you wonder and delight.

Life is more rich and generous when you do the work honesty invites.

Courage and an inner knowing are both necessary to practice satya, and qualities that are greatly cultivated and strengthened by dedicating yourself to living your truth and practicing yoga.

A Personal Account

When I was young, I was tremendously concerned with what people thought about me. Yet, my insecurities and sometimes-desperate desire to belong often repelled the very people I wanted to impress.

By trying to be what and who I thought they would like, I was denying my true Nature and making my own life quite difficult. The relationships I had at that time were fragile and false, for they were not built on the foundation of truth.

After many years of discovering the truth of myself, trying on personas and styles to see how they fit, I gradually chose to do the work necessary to be honest with myself.

A lot of that work was learning ahimsa (loving kindness), because to be authentic and honest with myself, I had to trust myself. When my self-talk was hurtful, there was mistrust. When that changed, little by little, I evolved into a confident, genuine, creatively expressive person.

I think this is a process that most human beings go through. It just takes some longer than others, which is perfectly fine because all things happen with Divine timing.

The Power of Truth

Though I have first spoken about being honest with yourself, this practice is, of course, a powerful and incredible influence on how you can relate to and experience everything around you.

One very beautiful expression of satya is how you know truth when you see it. It resonates with you when you feel it. You recognize truth when you hear it or read it.

There is an inner knowing on a subtle level that informs you on every level saying, "Yes, this truth is indeed a powerful thing."

The same goes for that which is untrue. You recognize falsehood and it doesn't feel right. Sometimes you just "know," without any other clue, that something is wrong or off. This, your intuition, is the power of truth as well, for you naturally want to align with Nature, and Nature tells you when something is untrue and therefore misaligned.

When Truth is Hard

Often truth requires courage. It may be because you've recognized something inside of you that needs to be worked on and won't necessarily be easy to resolve. Or it may be because you've seen something sad or disturbing in the world around you that requires courage to acknowledge and, possibly, change.

The truth of reality—of what is all around us as life—isn't always pretty, and it doesn't always feel good.

This is where the lines of clarity can blur because we can say that it is true that wars are being fought; trees are being cut down; people are living in poverty, fear and starvation; and all kinds of other horrible things are going on in reality. This is, on a very real level, a form of truth.

And yet, it feels very wrong because so much of these situations are founded in peoples' actions that are false and harmful—people who are not living in harmonious relationship with the world in terms of ahimsa (loving kindness) and satya (truthfulness).

Sat, the first part of the word satya, represents "reality." It calls to what is real and true. It identifies what is.

So, yes, part of practicing satya is acknowledging reality in all of its beauty and ugliness, just as it is in this moment.

Yet, if you go into the deepest, widest, most powerful, and constant form of truth, you connect with reality in a different way. You see the wholeness of truth as the energy, the One consciousness, which pulsates within us all.

And that form of reality, the entirety of the grand picture, shows you that even the ugliness is somehow held in love and will eventually return to love as all things in time and space are ultimately dissolved.

Resting in this grand perspective of truth, in contemplation and meditation, choosing to look for the truth in forms of beauty becomes easier and you find you have the courage to accept What Is in all its manifest forms.

The courage and inner knowing of satya nurtures a quality of ahimsa (tolerance), which in turn brings you to a place of clarity that can not be found in denial or falsehood.

MATRIKA SHAKTI: SPEAKING YOUR TRUTH

When you adopt satya as a way of life, how you speak becomes a powerful practice.

Why? Well, because words hold incredible force.

Sutra 2.36: satya-pratishthayam kriya-phala-ashrayatvam

Satya	truth, sincerity, genuine honesty
Pratisthayam	well established in, being grounded in
Kriya	action
Phala	results
Asrayatvam	dependence, foundation

This sutra tells you that when you are completely grounded in the practice of truthfulness, your words become potent to the point that what you say comes to be.

Yet not all words need to be spoken. Just because you honestly feel a certain way doesn't mean it's necessarily skillful to say it out loud . . . That can be a tough practice, I know, but this calls again to ahimsa (loving kindness) to help you choose the path of integrity.

It's always a good idea to pause before you speak and consider **The Four Gates of Speech:**

> *Is it truthful?*
>
> *Is it necessary to say?*
>
> *Is it the appropriate time?*
>
> *Can it be said in a kind way?*

Matrika Shakti describes the power of your words. The more mindful and truthful you are when speaking, the more powerful your words become.

Satya as Truth in Pulsation

To be sure that satya doesn't get dogmatic or static, I offer you this . . .

It seems to me, in my construct of reality and the constantly changing cycles of who I am as a person, that there are very few absolute truths compared to the infinite relative truths.

What I mean is this: something can be true for me and not true for you.

My truth and that of others is not always the same. For example, there are as many paths to God as there are seekers, yet some claim they have The One True Path. Though this is very real and true for them, it is not my truth because I follow my own path. No judgment is necessary here; in fact, it's a lovely example of how each person's perspective and personal truth leads us to the absolute truth of one conscious energy.

As well, something that was true for you or me last year (or month or week or hour, for that matter) may not be true for you or me now in this moment.

Seeking Truth

One name my Dragon uses is Seeker of Truth. In fact, I often use this as one of my own names because it describes me perfectly.

Truth invites us to seek it, to feel it, to align with it and to express it.

Satya is the practice of living in honesty to the best of your ability, and drawing on all of your skill to refine and expand how you experience life as a genuine person, authentic to who you are.

May this practice be a joy for you, unfolding mysteries and wonders of truth with your faithful companions, courage and inner knowing.

May you speak and live your truth with great beauty and delight!

Asteya: Owning Your Experience

Asteya, the third of the yamas as defined in the *Yoga Sutras of Patanjali*, translates as "non-stealing." Yep, you've heard it before: "Thou shalt not steal." Got it. Pretty common sense, right?

But that's just the tip of the iceberg: this isn't just about not taking what isn't yours but also knowing what is.

Sutra 2.37: asteya-pratisthayam sarva-ratna-upasthanam

Asteya	non-stealing, non-misappropriation
Pratisthayam	well established in
Sarva	all
Ratna	gems, precious things, wealth
Upasthanam	approaches, comes up

This sutra shows that the rewards of honesty in ownership are fruitful.

> *One who is trustworthy, because he does not covet what belongs to others, naturally has everyone's confidence and everything is shared with him, however precious it might be.*
>
> —Translated by T.K.V. Desikachar

Taking this concept a step further, by being aware and appreciative of what you have, both materially and on many other levels including your own unique talents, you realize how wealthy you are and embrace the many faces of abundance. When you're focusing on what others have, you enter a mentality of "there's never enough."

By seeing what is good in your life, you naturally adopt an outlook of gratitude, and you realize you have all that you truly need.

That doesn't mean that's all you ever get, or even all you want. However—and you likely know this from experience—if you're constantly wanting more, it is very difficult to be happy with what you've got, and the dreaded "never enough" feeling can descend.

And that's no fun.

So I like to think of asteya as owning your experience: taking responsibility for what is yours and not taking on what is not, nor taking more than is necessary.

This also includes not unbalancing our bodies or our planet by taking more than is right from any one part or resource.

How Asteya Can Help You Stop Worrying

For me, the hardest things to leave be as "not mine" aren't all the shiny toys and amazing clothes I'd love to own.

What I have a hard time "not stealing" are the feelings and perspectives of others.

With ideas, if they are borrowed, it's easy enough to give credit and honor the source as that idea is shared.

It's the judgments, worries, and feelings of others that are sometimes difficult to leave be.

Basically, "It's not my stuff; it's someone else's." But that doesn't mean I don't sometimes take it upon myself to try to fix or settle.

Here's a classic example: As a young woman I was very affected by how people judged me. But their thoughts of me weren't my choice; those thoughts were theirs. Not my issue, but I'd stress myself out about it all the same.

I still sometimes find that I'm quick to "feel bad" or experience guilt if I think I've offended or upset someone, often making it up in my head when they thought nothing of it. Or maybe it doesn't have anything to do with me at all, but a friend is worried and I somehow choose to worry with my friend (as if that helps anything).

Not only does this go against the truth of the matter (going back to satya—truthfulness) and it's not particularly compassionate towards myself (ahimsa—loving kindness), but I'm taking on (and often making up silly ideas of) someone else's experience, creating unnecessary worry.

Silly me.

Asteya as Contentment within Honesty

When we can simply be content and honest with what currently is, we realize we don't have to take on more than is necessary.

When we respect the experiences and belongings of others as theirs, we also can have more respect for our own experiences and physical comforts.

When you are aware of your blessings and take responsibility for your own thoughts and actions, you own your experience. Which is actually a lot more enjoyable than taking on what isn't yours.

> *By learning to gratefully acknowledge All That Is good in our lives, to respect our own talents and accomplishments as much as we admire others', to value our time and to use our resources wisely—and by practicing these skills—the desire to have what is not ours is gradually weeded out. We begin to recognize that everything we really need we already possess . . . Truly embracing the enough-ness, the abundance of our lives, we become a much stronger, peaceful force for positive change in the world.*
>
> —Margaret Huff

Brahmacharya: Unconditional Love and Highest Integrity

Brahmacharya, for me, is the yama that has changed the most in my understanding over the years. It went from being a concept that felt harsh and limiting into something that now inspires a deep sense of awe for me.

Why so, you ask?

Well, first let me introduce the concept of uttanita. You know it already, even if you don't recognize it by this Sanskrit word.

Uttanita is about shifting your perspective. It means "wide open; an expanded view."

You know it as the way you can take something you already know, turn it around, and see it in a completely different light.

And when this happened to me with brahmacharya I was delighted.

See, brahmacharya was first introduced to me as the practice of chastity, which really didn't really seem like much fun or at all realistic unless I were to crawl into a cave or retire to an ashram. Not that there's anything wrong with seclusion and the life of a monk or renunciate, it's just not for me.

Of course, the idea of restraint goes further than this, but I got stuck on the word *chastity* and couldn't see past it to the rest of what the teachings have to say.

Unsurprisingly, brahmacharya as an ethical practice of sexual restraint was a big turn off, and so I didn't really think much of it because I didn't feel it had anything liberating or positive to offer me.

Sexuality just didn't seem like a healthy area of my life to create oppressive rules around. Healthy boundaries, yes, but "restraint" or "chastity?" Not so much.

This is especially true because I had a hard time as a young woman getting through the confusing misconceptions surrounding sexuality in society. And I know I'm not the only one who grew up with low self-esteem and a great deal of confusion about sex.

But then came the uttanita.

Sex and Tantra

Before we get into the Aha! Moment that came as my new understanding of brahmacharya, let's first get the whole "sex and Tantra" discussion clear.

Tantra . . . Isn't that some practice of sacred sexuality? This is a common perception of Tantra. In a way, yes, that's true.

And yet, Tantra is much more than this.

Tantra is a non-dual philosophy, which means it comes from the premise that everything is a part of one conscious energy that manifests as infinite forms and experiences.

If you look at the world this way, seeing that everything comes from the Divine and IS an embodiment of the Divine, then sexuality is an expression of the Divine. That means it can't be classified as evil or only for the purpose of procreation because it can be an experience of Divine delight.

And yet, in so many ways sexuality has been abused, condemned, used, glorified, and genuinely confused, leading to centuries of complicated issues around something that is a natural part of life.

Think about it: the many difficulties surrounding sex—including rape, unplanned pregnancy, disease, prostitution and promiscuity—could be resolved if the world's understanding and treatment of sexuality was brought into harmony and balance.

Tantra says that sexuality is something to be respected, enjoyed, and treated with the highest integrity, *just like everything else.*

It isn't that Tantra focuses on sex, but that it includes sexuality as part of the honored cycle of life. This perspective towards sex is part of what makes Tantra such a different paradigm.

So, now that we've established that Tantra isn't just about sex, but a philosophy that includes every aspect of life, we can move on . . .

BRAHMACHARYA THROUGH THE EYES OF TANTRA

To be fair, I'd like to start by saying that Classical Yoga doesn't necessarily limit the concept of brahmacharya as much as my initial reaction to it did.

However, the descriptions I read when I was first learning yoga spoke more about control than my rebellious mind wanted to accept.

But when I got the Tantric perspective, a broader conceptual understanding of brahmacharya, it suddenly became something I could aspire to.

What if we all were to go beyond the act of sexuality and adopt instead the idea of "Integrity in Relationship?"

What if we were to broaden the view and go Big Picture with this idea? It would at least untangle us from the often-messy world of sexual ethics, wouldn't it?

This was my Aha! Moment. This is what changed my view so much.

Sutra 2.38: brahmacharya-pratisthayam virya-labhah

Brahmacharya	integrity in relationship, continence
Pratisthayam	well established in
Virya	vitality, vigor, power, energy, potency
Labhah	gained, acquired, obtained

One way to look at this Sutra is this: When you conduct yourself in the highest, in total balance and integrity in relationship, you step fully into your own power.

Oh. So this isn't about sex?

Well, yes it is. But that's not all it's about.

Whew!

Brahmacharya as Unconditional Love and Highest Integrity

Brahmacharya translates and can be defined as "having ethical conduct like God." To walk and act as a pure-hearted Divine being is something that totally aligns with the practice of being a Dragon Rider.

Brahmacharya invites you to practice living with the highest integrity, relating to others with unconditional love, free of manipulation or selfishness.

What does it mean to you, to walk like God? What does it feel like to imagine yourself as a perfect expression of unconditional love, living with the highest integrity as you relate to yourself and everything around you?

It is this question that brahmacharya asks you to consider and then practice in the ways that are most life-affirming and appropriate for you personally.

Because, when you relate in this way of highest integrity, you gain the power and vitality that you would associate with someone who walks in the footsteps of every Master who has graced this Earth.

But it isn't the power that entices you to this practice, is it? It's the idea of living so purely, as an embodiment of love and the utmost integrity.

As I imagine myself living such a high ideal, I am inspired.

I hope you are too.

> On brahmacarya. "This word is composed of the root car, which means "to move",
> and the word brahma, which means "truth" in terms of the one essential truth. We
> can understand brahmacarya as a movement toward the essential. It is used mostly in
> the sense of abstinence, particularly in relationship to sexual activity. More specifically,
> brahmacarya suggests that we should form relationships that foster our understanding of
> the highest truths."
>
> —T.K.V. Desikachar, from *The Heart of Yoga*

Aparigraha: Living Simply

Aparigraha, the last of the yamas as defined in Patanjali's *Yoga Sutras*, is a subtle and incredibly freeing concept.

We'll explore aparigraha (non-clinging) as the act of Living Simply.

This isn't a practice of renunciation, although some express it as such. Instead, it is a conscious way of living finely, simply, without grasping . . .

It is living in the natural flow of abundance with great respect in relationship with what you have and that which is around you.

Sutra 2.39 aparigraha-sthairye janma-kathamta sambodhah

Aparigraha	non-greed, non-hoarding, non-possessiveness
Sthairye	steadied, stable, confirmed (*shta* = "to stand")
Janma	birth
Kathamta	how, in what manner, in what way
Sambodhah	knowledge from awakening

When you practice being unattached to things and naturally live in sensitivity to the whole; when you are steadfast in your respect of resources and relationships, you awaken into a knowing of how and why things are as they are.

I was sitting next to my teacher at dinner one evening and he gestured to his shirt, saying, "You have nice things, but you need to be ready to give them away at any moment."

Aparigraha encourages us to let go of the grasping, possessive, neediness that is at the root source of greed. It tells us that we are far more free when we don't accumulate things beyond what is necessary.

When we live simply, even if that is living simply in luxury, we choose to practice the freedom of non-attachment.

Why? Well, let's look at this example:

THE DIFFERENCE BETWEEN PAIN AND SUFFERING COMES DOWN TO NON-CLINGING (APARIGRAHA)

There is a difference between experiencing pain and experiencing suffering. Pain is sometimes brought by the sensation of change. It is a feeling that occurs which can be acknowledged and then responded to in the best possible way. Yet suffering is different: suffering is the struggle that is caused when we cling to something and don't allow the change to happen. Struggling is fighting the natural flow of life, or denying "What Is."

Suffering comes when we constantly want something to be different than what it is, whether that is wanting something we don't have, not wanting to let go of something when it is time, or resisting the inevitable motion of change.

For most of us, accepting change is a challenging practice, especially when someone we love dies or a major transition comes, requiring us to say goodbye to cherished companions, experiences, or objects.

Yet when we cling, we don't serve the person leaving or situation changing, and we especially don't serve ourselves.

In the case of losing loved ones, our clinging to them can actually make it more difficult for their souls to leave their bodies and find peace. Being able to let them go is a great blessing to them. Sure, there is pain and grief, but these are wholesome and natural feelings. Without the clinging, we can go through the transition without suffering and can contribute to those souls' joyous freedom as they shift from this world into the next.

When anything in life changes, there is often pain, but we have the invitation to honor that which has come before by not clinging. Then we can flow with the newness, open to the next opportunity or gift given, and be in a state of inner peace and outer balance.

Aparigraha and the Environment

If we apply this concept of living simply and finely to our relationship with the environment, we can create a great deal of healing.

As a general rule, humankind has taken too much, too fast, and with too little awareness from this generous and beautiful planet we live on.

Instead of being a "throw away society," instead of consuming and even competing to have all the toys that our neighbors have, we can choose to live in ways that satisfy our desires and needs while at the same time living in right relationship with the Earth.

When we make choices that support sustainable living—like buying recycled paper products, eating organic and local food, and reducing our impact on the planet and its resources—we are practicing aparigraha. Much of this yama is about being mindful in how we acquire things and the impact our lives have on the world around us.

It's not necessarily a command to "not have material things," but rather it is an invitation to let go of the clinging of things as well as thoughts. This practice of non-clinging is particularly helpful in these changing times because it makes us less likely to struggle or fight against what is. . . and so we avoid suffering.

Here's another perspective:

> *The last yama is aparigraha, a word that means something like "Hands off" or "not seizing opportunity." Parigraha means "to take" or "to seize." Aparigraha means to take*

only what is necessary, and not to take advantage of a situation. . . . One who is not greedy is secure. He has time to think deeply. His understanding of himself is complete.

The more we have, the more we need to take care of it. The time and energy spent on acquiring more things, protecting them, and worrying about them cannot be spent on the basic questions of life. What is the limit to what we should possess? For what purpose, for whom, and for how long? Death comes before we have had time to begin to consider these questions.

—T.K.V. Desikachar, from *The Heart of Yoga*

I love Mr. Desikachar's translation of the sutra here. "One who is not greedy is secure." This is so true. When we stop clinging, grasping, and wanting, we feel centered; we feel free.

We can enter more deeply into meditation and understanding of ourselves and the world because there is nothing in the way. And since freedom is, ultimately, what we all desire, this practice is a beautiful way to move into and create it.

With this last concept, we will move from the yamas to the niyamas. Again, these are all guiding principles that we can use to experience more freedom and wonder in life: to live in right relationship, and therefore harmony, with the world.

Saucha: Clarity and Purity

Saucha is the first of the niyamas, and it invites great freedom through the practice of creating balance and purity.

While the yamas give us ways to live with high integrity and greater enjoyment in relationship with ourselves and the world around us, the niyamas are primarily focused on daily practices we do ourselves.

Saucha is a good place to begin when looking at your own personal practice, because it speaks to the importance of being organized and clear, and to the far-reaching benefits of cultivating purity internally and externally.

Simple examples: If your desk is a mess, how effective are you compared to when it is organized?

How do you feel when your house is clean and orderly versus when it looks like a clothing bomb exploded?

Fung Shui is a Chinese system of organization that places high importance on clearing out space and being precise in how things are placed.

For instance, if you've got a pile of unused and randomly stored "stuff" in the Wealth and Prosperity corner of your house, your Fung Shui consultant would tell you it needs to be dealt with in order to allow for full flow of abundance.

Hmmm . . . That sounds oddly familiar. Excuse me . . .

(30 Minutes Later)

Okay, I've cleaned out the corner. Energy flow clear. Ready and open for abundance!

SAUCHA: SPARKLING, INSIDE AND OUT

Really, this concept of creating clarity and purity in order to have more freedom and flow is reflected in every aspect of life.

Though the most important aspect of being clear and pure is that of your intention, the outside and inside always influence each other.

For instance, if the space you're practicing in is cluttered and dirty, sure you can still practice there, but the energy is different and not as clear. However, if you have a space that you keep clear, that you consider sacred, you will want to practice there more often and the purity of the space will absolutely resonate in your practice.

When you think about being pure, what comes to mind for you?

It may be that you think about the foods and drinks you consume. If they are wholesome and healthful, that shows in and obviously affects your entire state of well-being, including your emotional health.

Conversely, consuming toxins muddies mind, emotions, and body. It makes it much more difficult to enjoy and participate in life to the fullest.

Saucha not only invites clarity and purity in your surroundings and physical body, but also your thoughts.

I think this is one of the most important aspects of saucha. And yet, truly, they all fit together and support each other.

When you have a space that feels inviting and beautiful, it naturally uplifts your thoughts and emotions. When you eat good food and drink pure water, that vitality influences your thoughts.

And when you choose thoughts that are coherent, life-affirming, and that create balance, you move to a new level of purity that sparkles on every level of your life.

SO WHAT?

I always think it's a good idea to ask, "So what?" when dealing with any kind of life lesson. What's the why behind the principle?

This is sort of like me being a little kid who doesn't want to clean her room. "Why do I need to clean my room? What does it do for me? What's the higher purpose?"

In yoga, there's always a higher purpose, as well as an everyday application. In the case of the messy room, the higher purpose could be having a clear flow of energy, and the everyday application is being able to find what you're looking for because it isn't under a pile of other stuff.

The Universe is very orderly, even if that order is complex and we humans create chaos within it. When you look at the way life forms as a living organism, or how a galaxy spins, or how the seasons cycle, Nature is constantly showing us patterns and order.

When you create order and clarity in your life, Prana (life force) and Shakti (the energy or power of Nature) flow much more smoothly and happily.

Sutra 2.40: saucat svanga-jugupsa parairh asamsargah

Shaucat	by purity, by cleanliness
Svanga	one's own body (*sva*=self, *anga*=limbs, body)
Jugupsa	dislike, aversion, natural repulsion
Paraih	with others
Asamsargah	non-contact, non-association

This sutra states that when you practice purity in body and mind you align yourself with clarity and no longer seek superficial association with others.

> *When cleanliness is developed it reveals what needs to be constantly maintained and what is eternally clean. What decays is the external.*
> *What does not is deep within us.*
>
> *Our overconcern with and attachment to outward things, which is both transient and superficial, is reduced.*
>
> —T.K.V. Desikachar, from *The Heart of Yoga*

So what?

Well, by cultivating purity in each aspect of life, you are drawn more and more fully into alignment with that which is, and has always been, perfectly pure. You tend to the "outward things," and yet you lose your attachment to them.

This creates an enormous amount of freedom.

Practicing purity leads you into purity, and then, strong and steady in your own pure light, you can walk in the most defiled place and, just with your own vibration of coherence and clarity, shift it towards light and beauty.

Set your intention and align with purity and clarity, and they will become your experience.

Asana (yoga postures) and pranayama (breathing practices) are very much practices that cultivate purity and clarity when done with sensitivity and a life-affirming attitude. They are very potent ways to "clean house" on the internal level.

It's all about joy.

It's not just that you "should" clean your room so you can find stuff; it's for the pure joy and clarity of being able to look around and realize that your house (your body) is sacred, and that there is a purity that you have always had, and will always be yours. It's just that it is very difficult to reach when there is clutter in the way.

SIMPLE PRACTICES TO ENJOY THE FREEDOM OF SAUCHA

- ~ Keep your surroundings clear and clean.
- ~ Make a special place for your yoga practice, even if it also is used for other things. Keep it sacred, remembering that things can be sacred and functional both!
- ~ Keep your body clear and clean.
- ~ Eat wholesome foods, drink pure water. Eat moderately.
- ~ Traditionally yogis would bathe before practicing. Take care of yourself in manners that make you feel radiant and pure.
- ~ Practice yoga regularly.
- ~ Create rituals for yourself. Rituals instill order and precision because you do things a certain way and create a pattern of energy. Rituals can be anything really: meditating upon waking, blessing your food before eating, doing your yoga practice at the same time every day, taking a bath every Sunday night . . .
- ~ Focus your thoughts. When you catch yourself thinking something that isn't life-affirming or helpful, choose a different thought to replace it. You can also use mantra, such as Om Namah Shivaya, to turn your mind towards balance and clarity. Meditation and visualization can be very helpful in creating inner clarity that manifests and benefits your outer life.

Focusing on saucha can be quite motivating! I've cleaned half the house in between spurts of writing this portion of your Training. Possibly not the most precise way to organize when writing, but definitely a good thing for my house!

I hope you got some ideas from this that you can apply directly to your own life to create more clarity and freedom. Remember, a Dragon Rider sees clearly and knows without a doubt that the Divine is everywhere. When you cultivate clarity and purity you are a more effective and vibrant Dragon Rider.

Santosha: Deep Contentment

Yoga is a deep dive into the practice of equanimity, and santosha invites you to a level of contentment that is complete—a state where acceptance of the way things are creates a deep abiding peace.

The yamas and niyamas can guide the way to this state of peace and contentment, but it is your attitude as you practice and live that truly creates your experience.

And so, you each get to choose what kind of attitude you want to have.

Take my cat for example.

Jasmine, my rag-doll black and white kitty, has santosha down pat. Admittedly, her life is ideal for this practice as she really doesn't have any responsibilities other than being cute and cuddly, but not every cat has perfected the state of contentment like she has.

When I get too caught up in the "things to do," or the busy-ness of everyday life, Jasmine comes and sits on my lap, purrs, and basically says, *Chill out. It is what it is. Just breathe and be here in this moment with me.*

Wise cat, 'eh?

Here's the thing: when it comes to happiness, which is the goal of most human beings, santosha is the key.

WHAT DOES IT TAKE TO CREATE THE DEEP CONTENTMENT OF SANTOSHA?

It's all very well to talk about harmony and happiness, but how do you specifically create these states of being?

The first thing is to slow down for a moment and breathe; when you connect with your breath and the wisdom of your heart, you naturally move towards balance.

From this place of just pausing and being aware of the pulsing energy of life within, you can more easily choose to have an attitude of acceptance. You learn to adapt and approach whatever comes up with an outlook that is aligned with peace.

It's this attitude that informs your words and actions, so that's really the key to contentment. Pranayama, asana, and meditation are all incredibly helpful for moving stuck energy or emotions that get in the way of that peaceful attitude, as well as for creating a pattern where the attitude you choose becomes a habit.

When your default attitude is one of being centered in a perspective of peace and acceptance of how things are, you are practicing santosha. And you will naturally be a lot happier because joy and peace go hand in hand.

That's not to say that you'll never be angry, or upset, or hurt, or any of the other emotions that go along with being human. However, your practice of yoga can help you to be more balanced within those emotions—or, at the very least, not get stuck in them for too long.

Sutra 2.42: santoshat anuttamah sukha-labhah

Santoshat	from contentment
Anuttamah	supreme, unsurpassed, the highest
Sukha	joy, delight, happiness
Labhah	gain

This Sutra tells us that supreme happiness arises from deep contentment.

This brings to mind an image of Buddha, or the Dalai Lama, or a woman glowing with the spark of life growing within her, or a child who has just played an epic game of tag and is now lying on the grass gazing up at the sky.

Or my cat. She is happy because she is happy. There isn't any condition placed upon it, she just lives in a state of contentment because that is who she is.

> *The result of contentment is total happiness. The happiness we get from acquiring passions is only temporary. We need to find new ones and acquire them to sustain this sort of happiness. There is no end to it. But true contentment, leading to total happiness and bliss, is in a class by itself.*
>
> —T.K.V. Desikachar, from *The Heart of Yoga*

I think it's important to note this difference that Desikachar points out.

Sure, you can create temporary happiness with retail therapy or by getting excited about something, but that isn't lasting. It goes away after the excitement wears off.

True happiness, however, comes from the inner attitude and state of contentment—from acceptance of the way things are.

Dragons are pros at this.

> *. . . . Santosa, modesty and the feeling of being content with what we have. Often we hope for a particular result to ensue from our actions, and we are just as often disappointed. But there is no need to despair—rather, we should accept what has happened. That is the real meaning of santosa—to accept what happens. A commentary on* the Yoga Sutra *says: "Contentment counts for more than all sixteen heavens together." Instead of complaining about things that go wrong, we can accept what has happened and learn from them.*
>
> —T.K.V. Desikachar, from *The Heart of Yoga*

So, the more you flow with life, in acceptance, allowing each moment to be as it is and looking at it from a place of equanimity, the happier you are.

It's a practice of the kind of attitude and perspective you choose to adopt.

And when you forget, just think of my cat Jasmine, or think of your Dragon in a state of deep repose. Content wherever they happen to be.

Tapas: Discipline Serving Delight

Tapas could be thought of as the "fire of alchemy."

And, of course, your Dragon breathes fire, so you can do a lot with tapas.

Yoga gives you so many ways to tap into the powers of transformation, and tapas is a powerful force that can propel you to the next level . . . whatever that is for you.

Tapas asks you to transform your practice, and by doing so, yourself, with the purifying heat of willpower and intent.

In one sense, tapas is a very physical action of cleansing the body through the heat of practice and skillful choices about how you eat, how you breathe, how you're sitting right now as you read this . . .

And yet the concept of tapas goes far beyond the physical into your entire being as the liberating idea of "discipline serving delight."

> *It may help to ask yourself the following questions, to really reach into the depth of your motivation and dedication to your practice:*

How much do you want whatever it is you want?

How much do you want to be happy and content in your heart?

How much do you want to be free from pain in your body?

How completely do you desire to live with the highest integrity and joy?

When you meet that deep yearning with an equal amount of effort and dedication, the results are tremendous!

Discipline Serving Delight

Ah, discipline. The word conjures up many images and emotions. For the longest time, the idea of discipline equated to punishment and repression for me.

What is your initial reaction to the word *discipline?*

One of the great things I appreciate about yoga is how often it gives me a chance to change my perspective on things.

Not only *can* discipline serve delight, but to be balanced discipline *must* serve delight. If discipline is forced, dry, or joyless, then it is a form of violence, which goes against the very first yama: ahimsa (non-harming).

How can discipline serve delight?

By making possible that which you desire. Take this in the context of your deepest desire, or the highest wish of your soul.

Disciplining your body to hold a yoga posture longer increases your endurance and capacity to focus. Choosing to refrain from certain foods or from overeating can be a discipline that helps you be healthier. Introducing discipline to your speech can make your words more precise and powerful.

You can do any of the things above in ways that are helpful or harmful, depending on your intention.

For example: If you stay in a posture longer than is safe for your body, you risk injury. However, if you push your boundaries with awareness and self-honoring, your practice becomes stronger and deeper, bringing more bliss.

It's all in the motivation. If your intention is from your heart, discipline humbly serves delight.

TAPAS IN ASANA: PRACTICING ALCHEMY ON THE MAT

When you bring intensity to your asana practice it creates heat. You sweat. You invoke the fire of tapas by literally raising your temperature.

How is heat created? *Friction.*

Can you increase the intensity of your practice without losing the Big Picture?

Can you bring more will and fire to your mat so that, by moving through the challenge, you create a purifying action that is both physical and also goes beyond?

Of course, you can. You just do it in the way that is best for you.

Need more transformational heat? Just call on your Dragon . . .

How do you know if you've gone too far?

If your breath is forced or held, if the integrity of your alignment dissolves, or if you lose sight of the highest meaning, then the discipline is to back off, to pause; to begin again.

Alchemy is the transformation of one thing into another, using heat and purification.

Your Dragon can teach you a lot about alchemy.

Alchemy describes the physical act of purification and transformation, and also the philosophical process of rising above, of expanding into oneness—of crossing the threshold of the gateway of the heart.

> *Alchemy is an influential philosophical tradition whose early practitioners' claims to profound powers were known from antiquity . . . In general alchemists believe in a natural and symbolic unity of humanity with the cosmos.*
>
> —From Wikipedia

Interestingly, the practice of yoga, like alchemy, leads to legendary powers and cultivates the experience of unity. Thus it is a perfect way to train as a Dragon Rider.

The yamas and niyamas are in place so that those who actually achieve the superhuman abilities of the great yogis and Riders don't blow it by abusing their power.

Sutra 2.43: kaya indriya siddhih asuddhi-ksayat tapasah

Kaya	body
Indriya	senses
Siddhih	power, attainment of superhuman ability
Ashuddhi	impurity
Kshayat	destruction
Tapasah	self-discipline, passionate aspiration to attain perfection, deep devotion

This Sutra says: Deep devotion and self-discipline destroy impurities and bring Divine perfection and superhero-like powers.

The unity of humanity with the cosmos that defined the philosophy of alchemists sounds very similar to the aim of yoga, which is a conscious and integral union of Individual and Universal.

So, as you practice with heightened discipline, calling on the transformational heat of tapas, you can remind yourself that this is a practice that calls back to the roots of many traditions.

And it is up to you to direct your will, your disciplined efforts, toward the glorification of life, in service of Divine delight.

Your Dragon gives a joyful ROAR for that!

Svadhyaya: Deep Study of the Self and Yoga

"How far down the rabbit hole do you want to go?" asked the great (and humble) philosopher, Professor Douglas Brooks, in my first workshop with him many years ago.

"All the way!" I responded enthusiastically.

Sometimes I feel like I could just open up the top of my head and let the information pour in. When I am passionate about something, I study it intensely!

Of course, yogic texts can also be quite dense and hard to absorb sometimes.

I remember studying the Shiva Sutras as required reading for Anusara yoga certification. The text was so dense that, with the summer heat and the comfort of the couch on my front porch, I often found myself needing a nap every three pages or so.

Svadhyaya, the fourth of the niyamas, is a deep study of the self, through contemplation, practice, and also via the vast wisdom contained in sacred texts.

How to Study Sacred Texts

Let's jump straight to Patanjali's Sutra 2.44 and see what it has for us, shall we?

Now, when studying texts like this, there is an order to things.

First, try out the taste of the sutra before actually getting all intellectual. Say it out loud a few times and experience what it FEELS like, even if you don't know its meaning.

Go ahead. I'll wait. Repeat after your Dragon:

> "Svadhyayat ishtadevata samprayogah."
>
> "Svadhyayat ishtadevata samprayogah."
>
> "Svadhyayat ishtadevata samprayogah."

Next, break down the sutra into Individual words so you can formulate your own ideas about each one . .

Sutra 2.44: svadhyayat ishtadevata samprayogah

Svadhyayat	through self-study
Ishtadevata	chosen deity, patron saint
Samprayogah	communion, uniting with the Divine

Which gives you a pretty clear idea, doesn't it? Or maybe not.

The question is: What does it mean to you? Do you have any experience discovering a clearer connection with the Divine? Have you experienced a direct link into whatever you believe as truth in your heart through the process of self-study?

Very likely you have. Contemplate that for a moment.

After allowing yourself to sit with the feeling (*bhava*) of the sutra, and thinking about what it means to you initially and through your own experience, it's a great idea to see what others have to say about it . . .

Here are two different translations of the same sutra:

> *Self-study leads towards the realization of God or communion with one's desired deity.*
>
> —As translated by B.K.S. Iyengar

> *Study, when developed to the highest degree, brings one close to higher forces that promote understanding of the most complex.*
>
> —As translated by T.K.V. Desikachar

Generally those who translate the sutras will also give you more guidance as far as the meaning, for these small phrases can be unpacked seemingly infinitely.

Sometimes, to me, this is the most insightful part—you bring all of the above together with the perspectives offered by different teachers, and then you sit with it to formulate what it really means to you.

I quite like Desikachar's expanded ideas on the concept of svadhyaya:

> *Sva means "self" or "belonging to me." Adhyaya means "inquiry" or "examination"; literally, "to get close to something." Svadhyaya therefore means to get close to yourself, that is, to study yourself. All learning, all reflection, all contact that helps you learn more about yourself is svadhyaya. In the context of the niyamas we find the term often translated as "the study of ancient texts." Yes, yoga does instruct us to read the ancient texts. Why? Because we cannot always just sit down and contemplate things. We need reference points. For many this may be the Bible or a book that is of personal significance; for others it may be the Yoga Sutra. The Yoga Sutra says, for instance, that as we progress in our self-examination, we will gradually find a link with the Divine laws and with the prophets who revealed them. And since mantras are often recited for this purpose, we sometimes find svadhyaya translated as "the repetition of mantras."*

> —T.K.V. Desikachar, from *The Heart of Yoga*

Dive deep into the heart of self-study.

This is how you know yourself as a Rider and how you know the heart of your Dragon.

Use whatever speaks to you: meditation, asana, mantra, texts, and even seemingly random bits of songs on the radio, billboards, and fleeting encounters. All the elements of life can contribute.

And so, the question I invite you to think about is, "How far down the rabbit hole do you want to go?"

Every opportunity to study yourself and the world around you is an invitation to connect to the essence of All That Is.

And, of course, the more fully you know yourself, the more completely you will understand your Dragon.

Ishvara-Pranidhana: Deep Devotion and Joyful Surrender

Ishvara-pranidhana is the practice of total trust and alignment, or union, with the Divine, emanating a flawless faith that delivers you into complete connection and oneness of Universal and Individual.

It is utter devotion to the Divine, and absolute joyful surrender.

Your Individual self completely gives itself over to the Universal self.

And what happens is that, through this act of letting go, you experience a supreme wholeness and loving consciousness. This union is beyond description, yet so many have tried to explain this experience called Enlightenment, Nirvana, or Samadhi.

And this is what yoga leads you to; what all the practices are guiding you towards so that you can know yourself as a complete being, beyond the illusion of separation.

This is the difference between an Initiate and a Master Dragon Rider.

The Problem . . .

The problem most people face with devotion and surrender is that there are a lot of pre-existing trust and control issues.

These show up in myriad ways, but the fact of the matter is that when you have a hard time trusting yourself, others, or the course of life, things are difficult.

And when you look at the big picture, you are not, ultimately, in control. Yes, your intention, focus, and actions shape your experiences, but so do a lot of other influences.

So the answer to these problems is actually learning how to connect with and trust a higher power.

Of course, then you might run into sticky situations that have to do with religion and preconceived ideas about to whom and how you pray or connect.

My solution to this is to simply turn to the truth that resides in your *own* heart.

Whatever you call it—God, Goddess, Supreme Spirit, Universe, Divine, Creator—whatever name you give this conscious, omniscient, omnipresent energy, you already know it in your own heart.

And so, Ishvara-pranidhana says, connect with what you believe as true, as deeply and profoundly and completely as you possibly can.

Accessing the Ability to Surrender

There are many ways to learn to let go of the things that get in your way and interfere with your ability to access that all pervading oneness you're going for.

Here are a few examples:

- ~ Forgiveness (essential and incredibly powerful)
- ~ Lovingly identifying and intentionally releasing ideas and habits that don't serve your highest good and expression
- ~ Energy work
- ~ Journaling

And, of course, practicing asana, pranayama, and meditation.

These last three—the main practices of yoga—move and clear energy, support transformation and development of your awakened self, and help you tap into the part of yourself that is untarnished and eternal.

When you cultivate a connection to the Divine, you can trust the Universe to guide, protect, and nurture you.

This is huge.

And, really, it makes sense. When you surrender your worries and cares to a higher power, you are allowing yourself to be directed by a perspective and understanding beyond the scope of your Individual awareness, and in so doing, opening to limitless possibilities.

Sutra 2.45: samadhisiddhih Isvarapranidhanat

Samadhi	profound absorption, superconsciousness
Siddhih	attainment, spiritual success
Ishvara	God
Pranidhanat	by surrender, by complete devotion

Surrender to God brings perfection in Samadhi.

—B.K.S. Iyengar

This sutra tells us that the complete attainment of oneness and vast understanding comes from surrendering to the Universal energy that lives within you and all around you.

It is, and always has been, the ultimate practice.

When you align yourself with the truth in your heart, when your every thought, word, and action is devoted to this highest part of you and you trust that everything will work out in the best possible way (even when you can't see it at first), then you set yourself up for graceful transitions and successful adventures in life.

By dedicating yourself to this sacred and ancient practice of ultimate union, you align your thoughts, words, and actions in such a way that good things happen. Life becomes more beautiful, more flowing, and more joyful.

May you (and your Dragon) be blessed.

May your practice carry you through every challenge to see the gifts and growth each situation offers.

May you fly with the freedom in your heart.

May your devotion and ability to surrender joyfully bring you incredible insight, and may the positive results of your practice ripple out to bring harmony to everyone around you, and the beloved Earth who holds us all.

Integrating the Third Initiation

In order to complete this part of your Training and move on to the physical practice in the next section, you must set your intention to practice these Empowering Principles of Integrity to the best of your ability.

In every moment, you must be willing to do your best to live in right relationship with yourself and the world around you.

To be a Dragon Rider is to be completely dedicated to the highest integrity and to live a life that serves goodness, beauty, peace, and balance.

This is imperative because coming into your power carries with it the responsibility to wield that power as Light.

To make your commitment to the highest integrity, in a way that shifts the energies of the world and of who you are—to align with this pure purpose and intent—you may take the Oath of the Dragon Rider.

The Oath of the Dragon Rider . . .

To make this intention more powerful, to magnify it and to help you feel its meaning even in your bones, speak the following oath out loud and in a commanding voice.

Want to put even more power into it?

Imagine your Dragon standing next to you or behind you, adding its strength to your intention.

THE OATH OF HIGHEST INTEGRITY

I, _____, align myself with the highest integrity.

I choose to live in awareness of how my thoughts, words, and actions influence and create imprints in the manifest and energetic realms.

I live my life with these virtues of character to guide me in every moment:
- ⁓ Loving Kindness
- ⁓ Truth and Honesty
- ⁓ Respect and Honor
- ⁓ Unconditional Love
- ⁓ Simplicity and Flow
- ⁓ Purity and Clarity
- ⁓ Peace and Contentment
- ⁓ Discipline in Service of Delight
- ⁓ Deep Studentship
- ⁓ Profound Devotion and Trust
- ⁓ Service of the Highest Good

May my life be a practice dedicated to Mastery, in right relationship with myself and the world around me.

May the liberating effects of these practices benefit my own life and ripple out to uplift all around me.

May my life be an expression of skill, beauty, abundance, goodness, and happiness.

I, _____, willingly and joyfully align myself with the highest integrity.

And so it is.

You may also choose to create your own Oath here:

The Fourth Initiation:
Embodiment

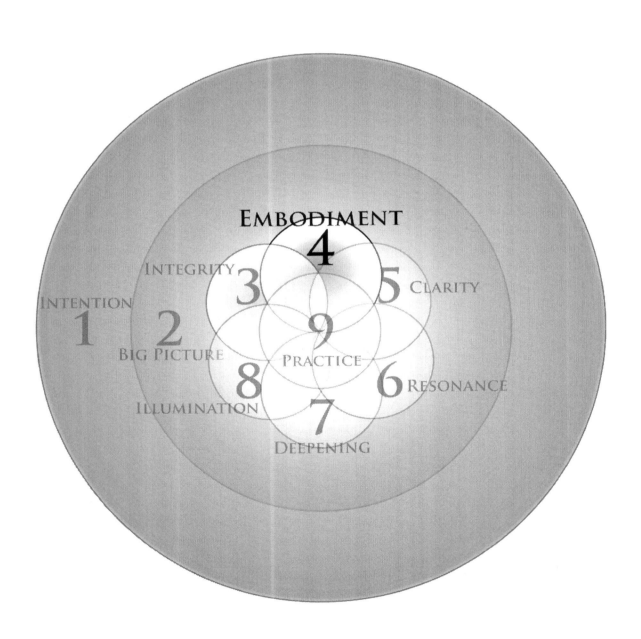

Breathe, Align, Move

ARE YOU READY TO RIDE YOUR DRAGON?

When you do yoga you move energy, which we describe and experience as Shakti.

Your mat holds Shakti, and that energy builds as you practice.

As you physically practice yoga and any other modalities of being in mindful, playful, skillful embodiment, you move Shakti.

You flow and co-create with the energy of life as you breathe, align, and move.

Your Dragon is an expression of Shakti, the creative force of the Universe.

So, as you practice yoga you are literally Dragon Riding, dancing with the Divine power of Shakti.

So, I ask again: Are you ready to ride your Dragon?

My style of teaching is Playful, Empowering, and Profound. Therefore, these are three of the elements you will notice yourself developing, from a vast scope of understanding and experience, as you practice.

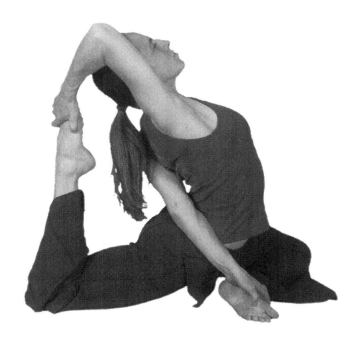

And, no, you don't necessarily have to do this pose. It's here for inspiration!
Eka Pada Rajakapotasana variation (King Pigeon Pose)

How we'll approach learning the physical practice of yoga in this Training:

1 – Learn about Asana
2 – Center In
3 – Learn Key Alignment and Poses
4 – Practice
5 – Close Your Practice

The Agreement

As we move forward it is agreed that:

You are completely responsible for choosing what is appropriate for your body and situation when it comes to the physical practice.

You will listen to your body and practice without forcing, straining, or going against your breath or inner knowing.

You are aware that studying in person with a highly qualified yoga teacher is essential for deepening your understanding and ability. You cannot always see yourself clearly, and a skilled teacher can help you progress much faster than you might on your own.

That settled, let's continue.

The Fundamentals of Asana

Breathe and Move into Balance and Bliss

The physical practice of yoga is comprised of different poses, called *asanas*. This is pronounced "AH-san-a," *not* "a-SAUN-a." A sauna is a small hot room you get into and sweat. Asana is a posture of yoga.

Practicing yoga on the mat combines the physical postures with mindful breath and intention. The asana practice is the most well known aspect of yoga, at least in the western world. You go to a yoga class to breathe and move, align, strengthen and surrender.

And, as a general rule, you always feel better after a yoga practice than when you started.

But it is of high importance that you know what you're doing. Like anything that can be of benefit, if yoga is misused, done in misalignment, or practiced without respect of what your body needs, it can create injury. Practicing with a highly skilled teacher is incredibly valuable to help you learn the best ways to approach yoga, and it is always key to listen to your body.

Say you're riding your Dragon—or practicing on your yoga mat—and you get an intuitive feeling that you need to back off or go a different direction. Obey that inner sense. Your Dragon—like your intuitive knowing—is incredibly smart and always has your best interests in mind. But it's up to you to be aware and take heed of those subtle signals that serve to guide your practice and life.

The following benefits are a sampling of a long list of why practicing asana is good for you:

- Releases tension and tightness
- Prevents injuries and improves body alignment
- Flushes out toxins in your body and scar tissue in your joints
- Improves strength, endurance, flexibility, and balance
- Increases lung capacity, circulation, and range of motion
- Improves concentration and reduces stress by using body and mind as one
- Great for balancing the body—very helpful for those who enjoy asymmetrical activities such as golf, snowboarding, and mountain biking (working on a computer and driving also count as asymmetrical activities)

Yoga, when done with skill and intention, benefits every single system in your physical body, including the cardiovascular, immune, nervous, endocrine, digestive, elimination, reproductive, and respiratory systems.

Good stuff, 'eh?

Practicing With Sensitivity and Awareness

The difference between stretching and yoga is the level of awareness that you bring to your practice. It is a dance of body and breath, heart and mind.

And so, knowing that this mindfulness is paramount to the practice of yoga, you first want to create a sense of spacious sensitivity and inner awareness before layering the elements of physical alignment.

A primary aspect of this mindful practice is being aware of and in tune with your breath. You'll learn more about breath in the Fifth Initiation, but keep in mind as you practice asana that your breath is your principal guide.

Here are some examples of different attributes you cultivate when you practice with awareness:

- ⁓ Freedom
- ⁓ Spaciousness
- ⁓ Receptivity
- ⁓ Illumination
- ⁓ Feeling of connection with Source
- ⁓ Happiness/Joy/Delight/Bliss
- ⁓ Peace and deep content

I think you get the idea. Inviting a sense of spaciousness and sensitivity first allows you to tune in to your inner being and the bigger energy that is everything in existence. And it isn't difficult to do. Your breath is always there to help.

Try this mini-meditation to increase your awareness:

Sit beautifully.

Settle into your hips.

Let your breath grow you taller.

Feel yourself be breathed.

Be spacious like a stainless sky.

Let your inner body be beautifully bright.

Soften your skin.

Notice the expansive feeling of being connected to something bigger than yourself, which naturally comes when you bring your awareness to the moment and turn to your breath.

Another great way to invite this sensitivity is to open your ears: listen, letting sounds come to you without grasping or judging, but simply witnessing.

SO WHAT DOES THIS MEAN WHEN APPLIED TO YOUR YOGA PRACTICE?

Well, first off it means you're not doing it alone. When you connect to a bigger energy you're not only more in the flow of the pulsation of your practice, but you'll find your capacity and ability is far more than if you were only working from your Individual mindset.

Also, by being spacious and receptive you are more able to receive the gifts of your practice—physically, mentally, emotionally, and spiritually. Insights can be more clear, and self-transformation more harmonious.

A NOTE ABOUT THE BREATH . . .

Though I'll give you more detailed breath instruction in the next part of your Training, it is important to note the following when you practice asana:

- ～ In general, breathe in and out through your nose. There are a few exceptions, and sometimes you just need a good sigh, but for the most part endeavor to do this.
- ～ Be very respectful of your breath. Breathe deeply without forcing or straining. Move with your breath, so that each movement you make is initiated by an inhale or exhale.
- ～ Make your breath smooth and flowing, rather than jagged or rough. Anytime you find that you're holding your breath, you've likely gone too far in a pose or you're thinking too much. Return your mind to your breath again and again.

Your breath is the bridge between all parts of you—mind, body, and spirit—and it is the force of transformation that allows all the benefits of yoga to happen.

Enjoy your breath!

The Importance of Foundation

Like any structure, yoga is built from the foundation up. If you look at an asana, or yoga pose, the foundation of the pose (the parts of your body that are touching the floor) affects everything else.

If your foot is placed even slightly out of alignment, it translates up to your knee, pelvis, back, and so on. If your hand is turned out or the fingertips are lifted, your wrist, elbow, shoulder and neck may have a few words with you.

Also, part of your foundation is an aspect of the Big Picture—setting your intention. By having a clear focus, it makes your practice more meaningful and therefore you get a whole lot more out of it.

Your intention could really be anything from simply wanting to feel more alive and free to longing to connect with your highest self and purpose. You can even devote the energy of your practice to supporting an area of the world that needs extra love, or pour your heart into a grateful practice dedicated to your teacher or loved one. Anything's game as long as it's life-enhancing, so get creative and let your heart suggest intentions for your practice. Notice how different your practice is when you make it more meaningful by using intention.

Having a beautifully aligned foundation is crucial not only physically, but also on every other level. When you line up your feet with awareness, it reflects and impacts your commitment to your intention. It makes it a whole lot easier to move into a place where your desire to feel good (or to realize any other intention) can happen.

Part of the skill you use in your foundation during yoga is based on your understanding of yoga, so it makes sense that everyone is at different levels. For instance, if I walk into a beginning yoga class and see that many of the students' feet are misaligned in warrior pose, it isn't fair for me to think that none of them are committed to their intention of benefiting from yoga when they simply don't know any better. But when I show them how to more skillfully align and they pay attention and apply that new knowledge, then *that* is a reflection that they are giving the practice their best effort, and that's a beautiful thing.

Conversely, if I have a more intermediate class and I've reminded someone nine times to keep her fingertips pressing into the mat in down dog, that person may need to make it more meaningful. She would do well to commit more earnestly to the integrity of her foundation and embody her intention to practice fully.

A Master checks their foundation every time because they understand how important it is. If you keep checking in with your intention and the alignment of the parts of your body that are on the floor, your yoga practice will be so much more rewarding.

The Pulsation of Yoga

The alignment and philosophical principles of yoga pulsate. This pulsation, in Sanskrit, is known as *spanda*.

When you do the physical practice of asana, you layer integration and expansion, always keeping the mindful awareness we just discussed.

You open, then you integrate. You expand and then you plug in. And you stretch out into the world in a way that glorifies the goodness of who you are and what your life is about.

Let's get a little bit more detailed in how these actions work . . .

Coming from a sense of internal spaciousness, you then strengthen your body. Your muscles embrace your bones, and you bring a safety to each pose by plugging everything in to your core. For example: if you are standing, without losing a sense of internal spaciousness, you tone your muscles and make your body subtly more compact as your arms and legs draw towards the center.

This integration serves to stabilize your entire body, including your joints, and helps you feel supported and capable.

To balance the strength and integration, you then stretch out. The key is to stretch without losing the integration. You're spacious on the inside, integrated through strength, and then you extend fully to express the pose. If we take the same example as above where you are standing mindfully, with an inner fullness and also a physical connection of strength, then—through the strength you have created—you also stretch out, extending into the ground through your feet and also up through the crown of your head.

Open. Contract. Expand.

Create spaciousness. Create integration. Stretch out!

In yoga we pulse between spaciousness and focus, strength and expansion, so that each moment guides you to further refine and delight. It is the balance of these opposites in cooperation that brings the feeling known as "yoga bliss."

The specific alignment of yoga is best learned directly from a teacher or with the help of videos so you can see the different elements in action. Yet, as you explore your yoga practice, just keep this idea of *spanda* (pulsation) in mind.

Everything in life pulsates. Even the molecules in the floor beneath you are vibrating on some level. Your breath is a pulsation, as are the cycles of night and day, the seasons, the tides, the beating of your Dragon's wings as you fly together, and the waxing and waning of the moon.

Yoga invites you to align skillfully, mindfully co-creating the pulsation of each asana.

And, of course, everything you do on the mat reflects in how you live off the mat . . .

Moving from the Inside Out

Just as you allow your breath to initiate each movement, so do you start with your intention. Your attitude permeates everything. That's why intention is so important.

When you have a "bad" attitude, or do a physical practice of any kind while focusing on negative feelings, those negative feelings are amplified. You might be angry or sad or feeling "off" when you start your practice, but you can shift those feelings just by *wanting* to. Set your intention to move towards love and happiness, and you will go there.

When you practice with kindness towards yourself and others, and are genuinely focused on finding freedom and feeling good as you practice, this is magnified.

So, first you set your intention.

Then you align to the best of your skill. You align your intention to the highest. You place your body mindfully, respectfully, and precisely.

You gather together all that you know, and then you take action and apply it.

You move and breathe. You make choices based on your intent, knowledge and skill.

Intention comes first, then knowledge, then action.

See how it comes from the inside out?

Moving from the Foundation Up and from the Core

Another key aspect of doing yoga from the inside out is the fact that you move from the foundation and from within to the outside.

You first align your foundation, whatever part of you is the base of the pose. Basically you start at the floor and move up.

You also move from the *core* of your body. The breath moves first, then the inner body, then the outer body.

For example, say you're in Triangle Pose. You would align your feet, legs, and pelvis. Then, as your breath moves, you unfurl the upper body, spinning from your lower belly up through the core, curling your heart and shoulders back, and *then* opening your arm up and stretching out from the pelvis through your legs, and from your pelvis through your heart, crown, and hands.

All this happens in the span of a few breaths. Wave by wave, the pose comes from the inside out with radiant expression.

Riding Your Dragon from the Inside Out

Imagine you are soaring high, riding your Dragon above the Earth.

How would you let your Dragon know where you want to go? First you'd have a feeling, which would turn into a thought; then you'd communicate that thought to your Dragon. Using its vast knowing of how to fly, your Dragon would realign itself in the direction of your choice. As your Dragon realigned, you would realign, too, by adapting your stance and gaze accordingly.

It comes from the inside out. From the wish in your heart and the knowing in your mind to the movement of your breath and body, all things come to be.

This is what yoga teaches you. This is what you practice on and off the mat as a Dragon Rider.

Centering In

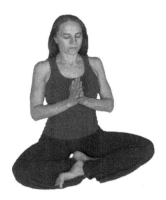

Every time you do yoga you first pause and center in. It can be a moment, it can be a meditation . . .

But in order to empower your yoga practice and align with your intention, you center in. This makes your practice more meaningful and shifts your state of awareness, bringing your focus to the dance of breath, body, and energy.

Centering in is an embodiment and enactment of opening to the Big Picture philosophy that connects you as an Individual to the Universal aspect of who you are. It also helps you set sacred space and be more present for your practice.

WAYS TO CENTER IN

It can be very simple, or it can be elaborate, but this ritual of centering in is essential to getting on your yoga mat and dancing with your Dragon.

You will find the best ways that work for you, and they will change depending on the situation.

All you need to do is attune to the Big Picture, and align with your intention.

SOME IDEAS:

- Take a few deep breaths and re-focus on your purpose
- Sit beautifully and meditate
- Om, or otherwise sing a mantra or invocation
- Invoke the feelings of gratitude, loving kindness, and peace
- Visualize yourself connecting with your Dragon, with crystal clear intent that your Dragon is an embodiment of your highest self in full Divine awareness.
- Invoke the feelings of awakening and delight.

When you move on to the sixth Initiation you will learn more about mantra and the power of sound, however, for now you should at least know the following mantras, as they are excellent ways to open your practice.

OM

What is Om?

When we chant Om we are tapping into a vibration that's already there . . .

Think of physics: everything, even to a molecular level, is vibrating, right? Well, one way you can think of Om is that if you added up all the vibrations of everything in the Universe, the sound you'd get is Om.

Om is the sound of the Universe experiencing itself. It is the sound of oneness, of unity, of being centered and at peace. It's the sound of pure joy and freedom. These are things we naturally want to align with as human beings.

When you sing Om as you hold an intention in your heart and mind, you literally bring that intention into the manifest world. Sound is the bridge between thought and experience. You can choose to infuse sound—in this case, Om—with meaning.

When you Om, simply notice what it feels like.

It is an invitation to feel your connection to something bigger, whatever it is that you already know as true in your own heart.

Om Shanti

Shanti is the vibration of peace.

Sanskrit holds the vibration of the thing it describes. When you chant the word *Shanti,* you enter into the essence of peace and can greatly shift the energy of yourself and your surroundings.

If you are ever in need of deep peace, such as when you feel anxiety, when you can't get to sleep, when you are upset, or when you are in a place that feels tainted, chant this.

"Om Shanti Shanti Shanti"
"Om Shanti Shanti Shanti"
"Om Shanti Shanti Shanti"

Even the reading of it makes this mantra begin to reverberate inside and out, bringing the vibration of peace.

It is a wonderful way to center in.

Key Alignment

The following section of your Training summarizes key alignment principles as they apply to the lower and upper body, which, of course, work together. The method I use is based on Anusara yoga's Universal Principles of Alignment™, which were developed by John Friend and are used by many top yoga teachers worldwide. This breakdown helps you focus and learn how to align in ways that are optimal for health and enjoyment.

It's nice to know that when you're riding your Dragon, you can lean into the turns and know how to respond to each nuance of flight. In asana, if your body gives you a signal that something doesn't feel good, this is important feedback. It's like your Dragon warning you that you're going to fall off if you don't shift your weight.

Knowing the optimal alignment for each area in your body—and how this alignment all works together to create an integrated wholeness—helps you to shift out of pain or discomfort, and can bring you into a more complete experience of freedom.

This alignment is also very effective therapeutically, so if you have an injury or any pain in your body, with proper application this alignment can speed healing and bring new strength. It helps you identify the misalignments that are creating the problem and then make a new habit so you can realign optimally for increased circulation and range of motion. Again, you might want a teacher to guide you through this in person.

It works like this: Healing occurs when you realign your body with its optimal design. This is the natural alignment of the body in its healthiest state, full of vitality—the highest potential of your Individual self, and your birthright.

When your body is in optimal alignment you have maximum range of motion, strength and stamina. Circulation flows, bringing nutrients and life into all areas, and all parts of your body work together as one. Thus, the body heals itself, which is what it is designed to do!

Key Alignment Principles: Lower Body Focus
(Lower Back, Hips, Feet, Ankles and Knees)

GENERAL ALIGNMENT
1. Mindfully place your foundation: Feet parallel, second toe mound in line with center of the ankle, knees facing forward. Stand tall, with your heart brightly lifted, head neutral, shoulders gliding back.

2. Spread and lift your toes:

Keeping the balls of your feet on the ground, lift up your toes and spread them wide. Distribute your weight evenly on the four corners of your feet (as shown here). Notice how this lifts the arches of your feet, and helps align your ankles.

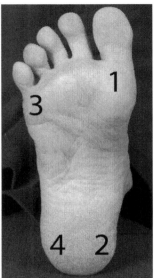

Lifting your toes helps to increase integration and strength throughout your feet and legs. Once you feel this engagement, you can stretch the toes and place them back down to increase space and extension.
KEEP THAT . . .

3. Shins Strong: Using the strength you just cultivated at your feet, DRAW YOUR SHINS IN toward the center. You'll also want to think of the base of the shin moving back, and the top of the shin moving forward to avoid hyperextending your knees. Knees point straight forward. Tone the muscles above your knees, especially those above the inner knees.
KEEP THAT . . .

4. Thighs Wide: Press your INNER THIGHS BACK AND APART—without letting your heels widen or knees roll in. You'll feel your pelvic floor widen and your lower back make more of an arch, emphasizing the natural curve of your lumbar spine.

5. Root to Rise: Keeping all of these actions, SCOOP your tail bone down and forward, and EXTEND from your pelvis down through your feet and also up through your spine and head—without letting your thighs pop forward or your pelvis tuck under. You should feel a toning in the lower abdomen and a feeling of spaciousness in your pelvis and back when you do this.

Observe your body in a mirror to look for patterns of alignment and misalignment. You also can try lying down to take notice of your alignment and move towards symmetry, feeling how one leg rolls out more than the other, one side of the back is more connected to the floor, one thigh is higher or lower, etc. This observation helps you increase your awareness, which will increase your ability to align your body in ways that feel good, on and off your yoga mat.

THINGS TO BE AWARE OF IN YOUR EVERYDAY POSTURE

Are you evenly placing your weight on all four corners of your feet?

Are your knees hyperextended? Do your ankles roll in or out?

Is your head neutral and heart lifted, or are you slouching?

Are you extending into the Earth from your pelvis so you feel tall and supported?

Key Alignment Principles: Upper Body Focus
(Upper Back, Shoulders, and Neck)

GENERAL ALIGNMENT FOR SHOULDERS AND NECK

1. From the inside (with your breath) INHALE and GET TALL AND FULL. On an inhale lift from your hips to your armpits and fill up with space in the front and back of your torso.
KEEP THAT . . .

2. With your THROAT OPEN (head neutral rather than tipped forward or back), take the HEADS OF YOUR ARM BONES BACK. You'll be using muscles to bring your shoulder blades more onto your back and strengthening the rotator cuffs by keeping the heads of the arm bones back. *Move them back from both sides: outer edges AND inner edges.*
KEEP THAT . . .

3. From the inside, BROADEN by extending from the center of your body out through your shoulders, arms, and crown of the head. This creates a lengthening and helps the alignment feel more natural. (To be balanced, remember that this entire alignment of the upper body is supported by the alignment we just discussed in the lower body).

THINGS TO BE AWARE OF IN YOUR EVERYDAY POSTURE

Is your head neutral?

If your head tips forward, it rolls the shoulders forward and lessens the circulation to your shoulders, neck, arms and wrists. Think about looking evenly out of both your upper and lower eyelids. You may also like the phrase "throat open," imagining a clear channel through the front and back of your throat physically, and also being sure to speak your truth—expressing yourself with confidence and skill rather than diminishing the throat chakra.

Is your heart lifted?

When you collapse your chest and slouch your back, your shoulders roll forward, your head will tend to fall forward, your breath will be restricted, and you are far more likely to have feelings of sadness, depression, frustration and the like. As soon as you lift your heart brightly, your attitude will shift towards happiness and it will be far easier to align your head and shoulders.

Yoga for the Wrists and Hands

It's important to remember that optimal shoulder and neck alignment allows optimal circulation to the hands and wrists. So do all of the alignment you've learned, and add the following to learn hand and wrist positioning:

Spread your hands on a table or yoga mat. You want to use the most weight bearing pose that you can WITH FULL INTEGRITY. That means that if you have weak wrists or injuries then you can start with your hands on a table so they have very little weight on them. Once you feel confident with that then you can start moving towards hands and knees, and then into Downward Dog on your mat. Just ensure you can do the following alignment fully wherever you're working.

Remember this is in sequential order, so your fingertips anchor a moment before the four corners of your hands, not the other way around.

1. Place your hands so the outer shoulder is even with the center of your wrists. This is how wide you want your hands for positions like Down Dog, Plank, and Cobra.

2. Align your wrist creases parallel to the top of your mat or the edge of the table. This way your hands don't turn in or out.

3. ANCHOR YOUR FINGERTIPS. Spread your fingers comfortably wide, and PRESS STRONGLY through all five FINGERTIPS. Claw the surface like a Dragon by allowing the knuckles in between your palm and fingertips to lift, but not the base knuckles where the fingers meet the palms or the fingerpads themselves. These stay firmly rooted and help you distribute your weight more evenly through your hands.

4. Press down through all FOUR CORNERS of your hand, especially the knuckles where your index fingers meet your hands (position 1 in the diagram). These ones are sneaky and try to lift up often. Don't let them, as keeping them down actually supports the alignment of your shoulders as well as your wrists and hands.

5. With optimal shoulder and head alignment, keeping your hands where they are, DRAW inwards to INTEGRATE your arms isometrically towards each other, and also towards your torso, gathering that strength and energy into the bottom of your heart and DRAWING your SHOULDER BLADES BACK by moving the head of the arm bones back. Feel your forearms, especially underneath, grow strong and stable. You should feel like the center of your palm is lifting somewhat like a suction cup.

6. From your heart, where you just drew into, EXTEND out through the bones of your arms through all four corners and five fingertips of your hands.

If you're using this therapeutically, you can hold this for 30 seconds, or start with less time if you are working with injuries and 30 seconds is too much. Rest and then repeat. Do this often, every day, and your wrists will strengthen considerably and quickly. This is what you use for Downward Dog or any time your hand is "flat" on any surface.

Quick Fix Yoga: For optimal alignment and circulation.

These two exercises are fantastic if you just need a pick-me-up or to open your shoulders and breath. You'll also get a nice increase in circulation through your spine, hips, legs, internal organs, chest, and shoulders.

If it's been a while since you've ridden your Dragon, or you've been sitting for long hours, these two simple stretches can make a big difference in how you feel.

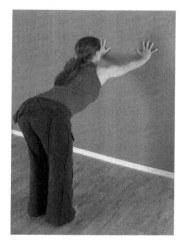

1. Forward bend at wall:

Practice getting the foundation set with precision, especially focusing on the four corners of your feet, lifted arches, lower legs strong and thighs wide.

From there, lengthen your torso using your breath, breathe your back body full, and take the heads of your arm bones back with your throat open.

Extend from your pelvis out through your feet and out through your hands. Be sure your lower back stays long, even if you have to keep your knees bent a bit.

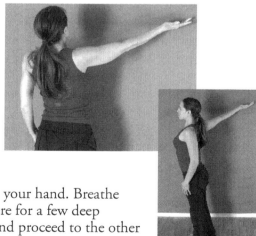

2. Shoulder/Chest opener at wall:

Palm faces up, body faces the wall. Set yourself up with the alignment we've just gone over, growing tall and taking your shoulders back with your breath. Then press the edge of your hand into the wall and turn your feet and body away only as far as comfortable.

Remember to extend from your heart through your hand. Breathe and invite increased circulation. Smile! Stay here for a few deep breaths, then inhale to come out of the twist and proceed to the other side.

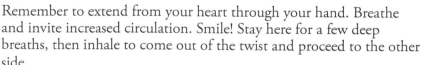

3. Repeat forward bend at wall.

Key Asana Poses

The following section includes some key poses and how to apply general alignment to them.

Asana is the Sanskrit word for "posture," literally referring to how you sit for meditation, as well as how you position your body in other ways.

If you think of the awareness and devotion with which you would sit if you were one with the essence of life, you'll get an idea of the meaningful focus you can also bring to the different postures you use in your asana practice.

By studying the descriptions of the following foundational poses, you can deduce how to apply the same alignment principles to the other poses included in the sequences of the next section. Working with these basic poses also helps you develop strength and stability. This is also nice in helping you respond skillfully when your Dragon does a loop-de-loop or a deep dive in flight.

Sun Salutation (Surya Namaskar)

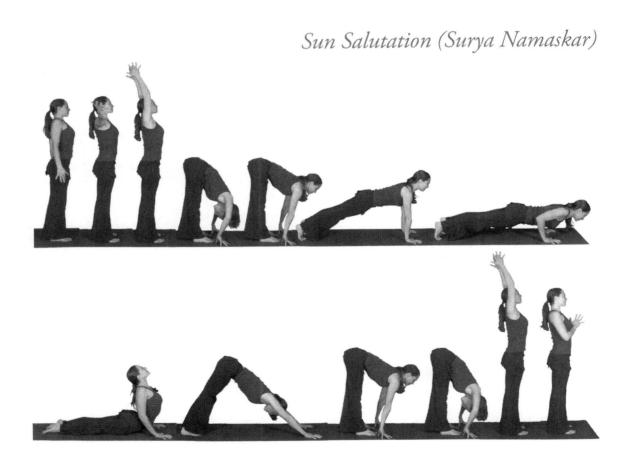

Surya Namaskar and Vinyasa (The Sun Salutation)

Significance: This is the main thread of yoga flowing through a series of poses found in nearly every practice. It honors the sun, the Earth, the cyclical Nature of life, and the pulsating practice of balance and harmony.

Benefits: Everything. Helps to clear, balance, and cleanse the palate. Particularly helpful as a transition. Specific benefits for each pose follow.

Key Alignment: The primary attribute of Surya Namaskar is flowing awareness in the current of your breath. Use all the alignment you know, and stay present.

This is also called Vinyasa, and when you see Vinyasa in a practice sequence it invites you to flow through plank, cobra, and downward dog (without the forward bend or coming to standing).

When you see this <VINYASA> you can add this flow to your practice, or a sun salutation, as you see fit.

Vinyasa Flow

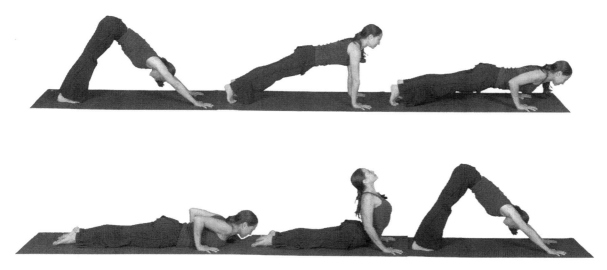

Tadasana (Mountain Pose)
Also known as Samastithi (Equal Standing)

Significance: Equanimity. Centeredness. Readiness. Stillness. Bridging Earth and Sky.

Benefits: Grounding. Helps you create balance and focus. Brings even awareness to foundation and helps tone the legs and core. A good place to pause, feel, and collect yourself as you practice.

Cautions/Modifications: If you are injured, in a wheelchair, or simply needing to refine your posture while you're sitting, you can do a seated version of this pose. Bring awareness and alignment to your body, allowing yourself to access the balancing benefits of this pose in a seated position, and open to your breath.

Key Alignment for Tadasana:

- Stand with feet parallel, and weight evenly distributed on all four corners of your feet.

- Spread your toes to tone your legs.

- With your breath, lift your heart and gently take your shoulders back.

- Draw power and strength up from the Earth into your pelvis, and then extend from your pelvis into the Earth and Sky.

Uttanasana (Standing Forward Bend)

Significance: Connecting to Earth. Turning inward. A humble bow.

Benefits: Calming. Stretches the hamstrings and calves. Can assist in improving digestion; relieving stress, anxiety, headaches, and insomnia; and reducing fatigue.

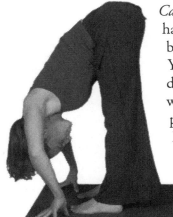

Cautions/Modifications: Keep the lower back long, not rounded. If you have a back injury or your hamstrings are tight and cause the lower back to round, bend your knees and/or use blocks beneath your hands. You can also do a modified version of this with your hands on a wall, desk, or chair; or step your feet wider for a wider forward bend (as wide as your mat works well). Modifying will help you access the pose and work towards a deeper forward bend when you are ready. Refrain from locking your knees if your legs are straight, instead use the muscles of your legs to straighten.

Key Alignment for Uttanasana:

- ~ With strong legs, feet parallel and slightly apart, touch the floor or blocks with your fingertips.

- ~ Without moving your feet, draw your shins towards the midline as you simultaneously widen your knees and spin your inner thighs back. Keep your lower back long.

- ~ Root from your pelvis through your feet, and extend from your pelvis through your heart and head. Be sure to keep your head neutral—avoid pulling your head forward. Enjoy your breath.

Variations for Uttanasana

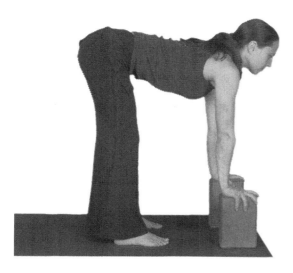 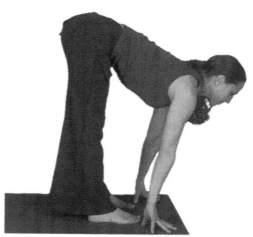

ADHO MUKHA SVANASANA (DOWNWARD FACING DOG)

Significance: Grounded. Connected. Playful. Balanced. Opening.

Benefits: Calming, energizing. Strengthens arms, legs, shoulders and hands. Stretches legs, hips, and shoulders. Improves organ function and digestion. Brings relief for fatigue, insomnia, headache, mild depression and anxiety. Helpful for balancing high blood pressure, toning the arches of the feet, relieving sciatica, and bringing relief for asthma.

Cautions/Modifications: If your wrists, hands, or shoulders hurt when you do this pose, try it at the wall as suggested in the last section. You can modify with Dolphin so it is not weight bearing on your wrists, or use Child's pose or Uttanasana as an alternative. Also, emphasize the alignment for hands and shoulders, which will help bring more circulation to these areas.

Key Alignment for Adho Mukha Svanasana:

- Align your hands precisely, outer edge of the shoulders in line with the center of the wrists.

- Start with your knees bent, especially if you have tight hamstrings—this allows you to keep your lower back long and NOT rounded up.

- Create space with your breath by lengthening from your hips to armpits, and draw your shoulder blades onto your back.

Down Dog

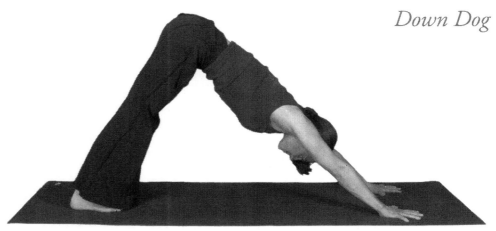

- As you integrate by drawing your arms toward each other, also draw your shins toward each other keeping your feet hip-width apart.

- Keeping your knees bent, send your inner thighs back without letting your knees roll in. Doing this creates space in your back.

- Keeping your lower back long and not allowing it to round up, scoop your tail bone toward your heels so you feel your lower belly tone and your lower back lengthen.

- From your heart, stretch down through your arms and hands, and from your heart, extend up and over your hips, down through your legs bringing them as straight as possible without letting your lower back round. (This means if your hamstrings are tight you might keep your knees slightly bent in Down Dog or Dolphin).

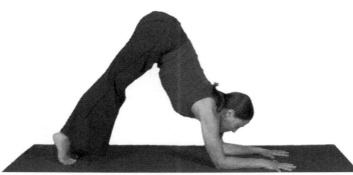

Dolphin

Chaturanga Dandasana (Four-Limbed Staff Pose and Plank)

Significance: Stability. Alignment. Strength in transition.

Benefits: Strengthens the whole body, including the core. Helps create a balancing effect between forward bends and back bends.

Cautions/Modifications: If your wrists prevent you from doing this, try forearm plank to build up strength. You may also take your knees down until you have cultivated strength and are ready for the full pose. If you need to modify further, you can try plank and push-ups with your hands on a wall to build strength gently.

Key Alignment:

~ In a plank position (knees raised or touching the ground), using optimal alignment for your hands, take a breath and lengthen your torso.

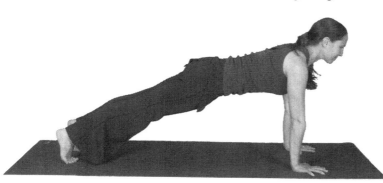

~ Hug the muscles of your body onto your bones, drawing your legs and arms toward the midline without moving your feet. This will create more stability and strength.

~ Draw your shoulder blades onto your back and keep your head neutral, not letting it drop down.

~ With the tops of your thighs lifted, scoop your tail bone toward the ground to enhance abdominal strength.

~ Extending from your pelvis in all directions and keeping your shoulders back, bend your elbows and, with an exhale, lower yourself halfway to the floor. This is Chaturanga. You can continue to the floor from there, hold for strength, or play with some push-ups.

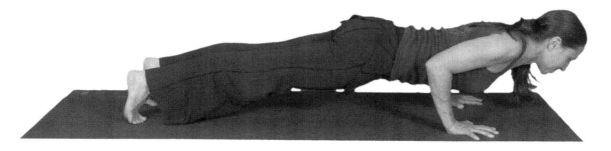

BHUJANGASANA (COBRA)

Significance: Anchored. Fearlessness. Revealing the splendor of the Heart. (Also, being a serpent and therefore cousin to Dragons, you can apply the appropriate metaphors as you see fit).

Benefits: Strengthens the legs, back, shoulders, arms and spine. Stretches the abdominals, chest, and fronts of the shoulders; expands the lungs. Helps bring relief from fatigue, depression, and stress. Lightens and benefits the heart.

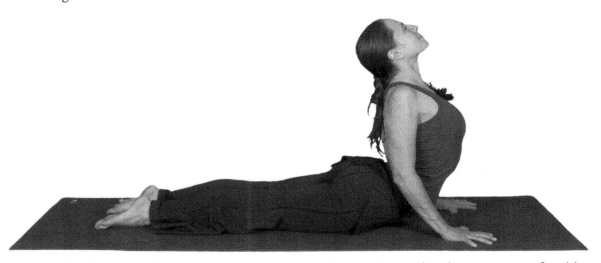

Cautions/Modifications: If you have a back or wrist/hand injury that makes this pose uncomfortable, try Sphinx pose instead with your elbows under your shoulders and your forearms on the floor. If you are chair-bound, do a gentle seated backbend with your hands on the chair's arms. Lift with your breath from the inside, keeping your pelvis and legs anchored, and then curl back as far as it feels good. If pregnant, you can modify by arching your back on your hands and knees, or placing your thighs on a bolster to keep your belly off the floor.

Key Alignment:

 - Lying on your belly with your hands near your ribs, spread your fingers and press the pads of your fingertips down. Strengthen your legs.
 - Lengthen, from the inside, so that your heart draws forward.
 - Claw your finger pads into the floor and bring the heads of your arm bones (shoulders) toward the sky, curling up and back with an inhale.
 - Scoop your tailbone toward the Earth and press your legs down as you reach your heart forward and continue to curl your shoulders back.
 - Keep space in the front and back of your throat, even if you take your head gently back.
 - Stay for a breath or several breaths, exhale to lower down. Transition into Down Dog.

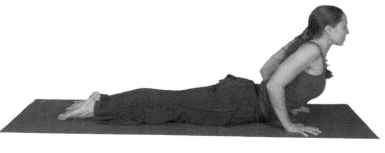

Low Cobra

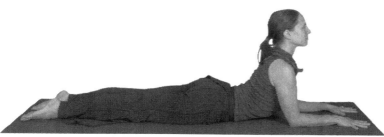

Sphinx

VIRABHADRASANA I (WARRIOR I, CRESCENT VARIATION)

Significance: Courage. Balanced strength. Foresight. Celebration.

Benefits: Strengthens the whole body. Stretches the legs, hip flexors, chest and shoulders. Increases balance and stamina.

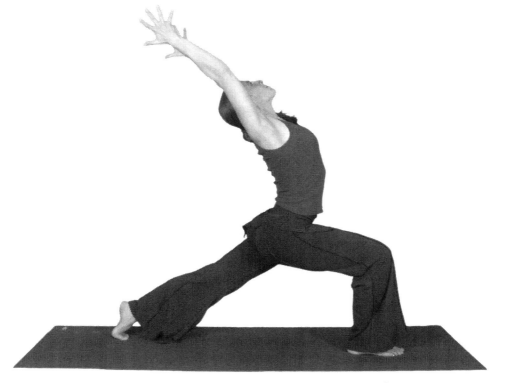

Crescent Lunge

Cautions/Modifications: If you have high blood pressure or a heart condition, you may need to keep the arms below your shoulders or gradually work up to this pose. You can also take your back knee to the floor, or do this pose with your hands against a wall for more support.

Key Alignment:

- ~ Note: While you are learning, do this pose with your back heel lifted, as it requires more refined alignment to take your heel down.
- ~ With feet, legs and hips square to the front, bend your front knee over your ankle. Be sure your knee points toward the second and third toe, and that it doesn't roll in or out. Ideally, you want a 90-degree bend in your front leg.
- ~ Strengthen your legs and draw strength up from your feet to your pelvis.
- ~ Lift your back thigh, and then reach your tailbone towards your front knee and draw your outer hip down on the front leg.
- ~ Extend from your pelvis through your feet into the Earth and inhale to float your arms up to the sky, heads of the arm bones back.
- ~ With each breath, get brighter, feeling your back hip flexors and thigh stretch and open.

left: *Anjaneyasana* . . . center: *Warrior I* . . . right: *Lunge variation*

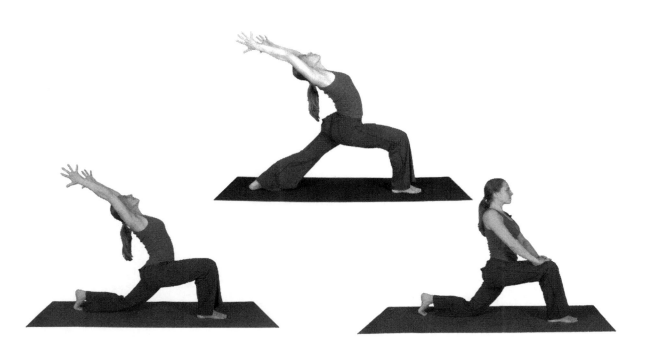

Virabhadrasana II (Warrior II)

Significance: Valor. Steadfastness. Bravery. Honoring past and future while steady in the present moment.

Benefits: Builds strength and stamina. Stimulates internal organs. Stretches the groins, chest and shoulders.

Cautions/Modifications: If you have high blood pressure, you may need to keep your hands on your hips or build up to this pose slowly to increase stamina as your blood pressure is regulated. If you have injuries that make this pose difficult, you can shorten the stance or do the pose sitting on a chair.

Key Alignment:

- Take a wide stance, measuring so that your ankles are under your wrists when your arms are out to the sides. Turn one foot outward. Your feet should line up so that the front heel is in line with the back arch, and your feet are parallel to their respective sides of the mat (front foot parallel to the long side, back foot parallel to the back of your mat).

- With an inhale, lift your arms out and create space inside. Exhale to bend your front knee directly over the ankle. Be sure your knee points toward the second and third toe, and that it doesn't roll in or out. Ideally, you want a 90-degree bend in your front leg.

- Spread your toes, make your legs strong and draw energy up from your feet into your pelvis. Draw from your hands into your heart, with your shoulder blades coming onto your back.

- Spin your inner thighs back, especially the straight leg thigh. Keeping that, scoop your tailbone down and forward while you tack your outer hip down on the front leg.

- Stretch out, extending from your pelvis down through your feet into the Earth, and from your pelvis up and out through your arms and head.

- Keep your torso centered, rather than leaning to one side. Turn your head to look at your front hand only if it feels natural for your neck. Breathe.

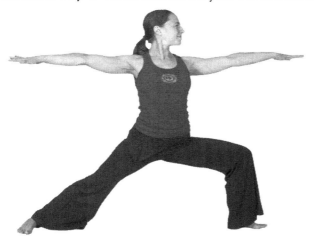

Warrior II

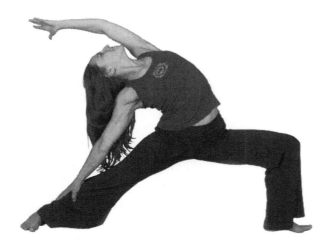

Utthita Parsvakonasana (Extended Side Angle Pose)

Significance: Flexibility and ability to be aware and have influence on many levels at once. Clarity in multitasking.

Benefits: Strengthens and increases stamina. Stretches the groins, hips, side body, shoulders and chest. Stimulates and cleanses the internal organs.

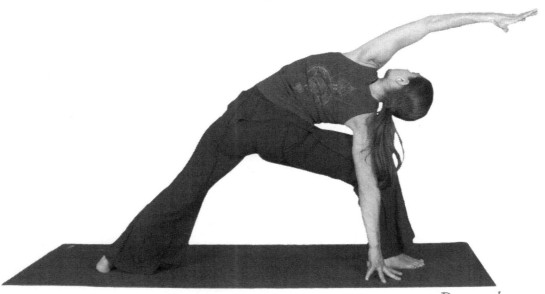

Parsvakonasana

Cautions/Modifications: You may need to work up to this pose if you have high or low blood pressure. You also may want to keep the top hand on your hip rather than raise it in the air. To modify, do the pose with your forearm on your thigh. If you need more support, do this pose sitting on a chair or with your front hand on a chair.

Key Alignment:

~ Take a wide stance, measuring so that your ankles are under your wrists when your arms are out to the sides. Turn one foot outward. Your feet should line up so that the front heel is in line with the back arch, and the feet are parallel to their respective sides of the mat (front foot parallel to the long side, back foot parallel to the back of your mat).

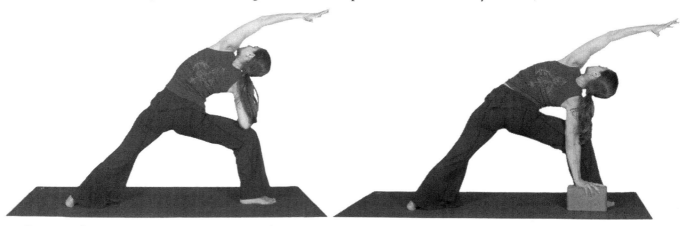

Parsvakonasana Variations: forearm on thigh and with a block

~ With an inhale, lift your arms out and create space inside. Exhale to bend your front knee directly over the ankle. Be sure the knee points toward the second and third toe, and that it doesn't roll in or out. Ideally, you want a 90-degree bend in your front leg.

~ Spread your toes, make your legs strong and draw energy up from your feet into your pelvis. Draw from your hands into your heart, with the shoulder blades drawing onto your back.

~ Take your front forearm to your thigh, or place your fingertips on the floor or a block. Take your top hand to your hip or ribs.

~ Spin your inner thighs back, especially the straight leg thigh. Keeping that, scoop your tailbone down and toward your front knee while you tack the outer hip down on the front leg.

~ Stretch out, extending from your pelvis down through your feet into the Earth, and from your pelvis up and out through your arms and head.

~ Using your breath, lengthen and extend your torso—from your lower belly upwards—spinning your heart towards the sky.

~ Take your shoulders back, then inhale to reach your top arm up and over your head, upper arm by your ear.

Utthita Trikonasana (Triangle Pose)

Significance: Connection to Earth, sky and stars. Powerful presence. Fortitude. Acceptance. Balance of strength and surrender.

Benefits: Strengthens and increases stamina. Stretches hamstrings, groins, hips, side body, shoulders, chest and spine. Stimulates and cleanses internal organs, improving digestion. Helps relieve back pain, stress, anxiety, and sciatica.

Cautions/Modifications: If you have high or low blood pressure, you may want to work up to this pose or modify, keeping the top hand on your hip. You can do the pose with a wall behind you, or put your bottom hand on a chair. Be careful that you don't hyperextend or lock the knees, instead use the muscles above the kneecaps to lift and strengthen.

Key Alignment:

- Take a wide stance with your feet aligned to the center and parallel to their respective sides of your mat. Front foot turns out.
- Bend your front knee and touch the floor with the same side hand. Use a block if your hamstrings are too tight. You can also come into this pose from a low lunge.

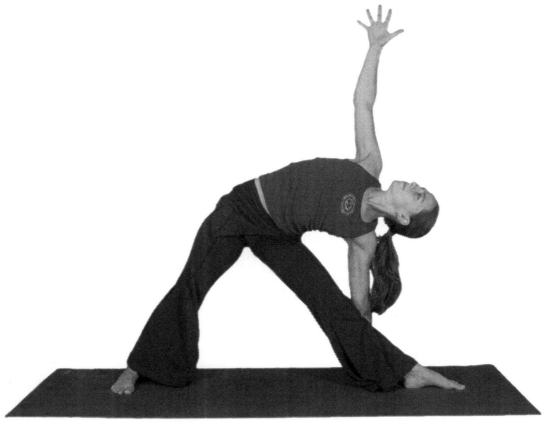

Trikonasana (Triangle Pose)

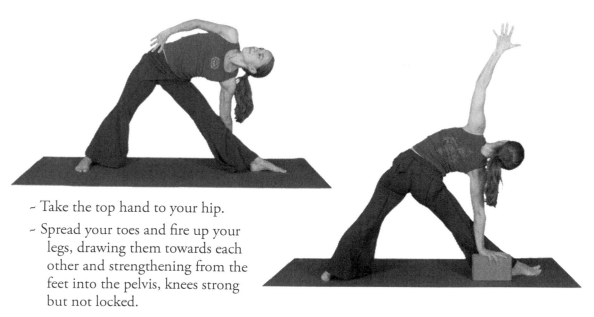

~ Take the top hand to your hip.

~ Spread your toes and fire up your legs, drawing them towards each other and strengthening from the feet into the pelvis, knees strong but not locked.

~ Keeping the strength, send your inner thighs back, even exaggerating and sticking your butt out. The tops of the femurs move deeper into the hip sockets.

~ Keep that, and then scoop your tailbone down and front hip under so your front knee points towards the second and third toes of that foot.

~ Extend from your pelvis into your feet and from your pelvis through your torso. With your breath lengthen your spine and twist upwards gently.

~ Coming back from your shoulders, heart, and head, extend your torso and brightly reach your top hand to the sky. Enjoy your breath.

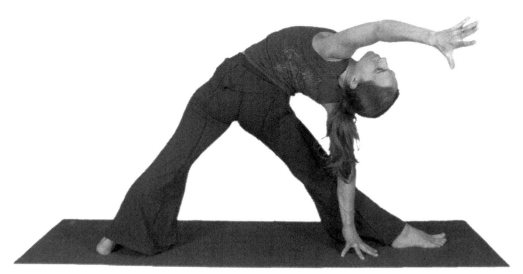

Trikonasana backbend

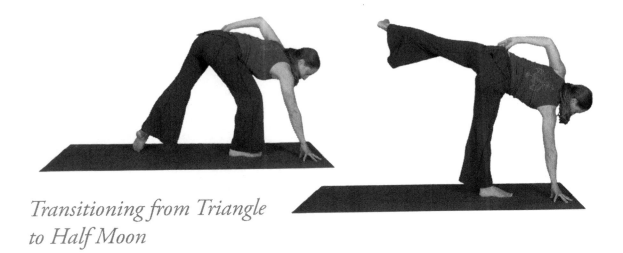

Transitioning from Triangle to Half Moon

ARDHA CHANDRASANA (HALF MOON)

Significance: Balanced perspective. Open awareness. Playfulness. Willingness. Sensitivity.

Benefits: Strengthens and improves balance. Improves digestion and tones the reproductive organs. Stretches the hamstrings, groins, chest, spine and shoulders.

Cautions/Modifications: Transition slowly if you have low blood pressure. You can do this pose with a wall behind your back or with your raised foot against it. You can also place your bottom hand on a block or chair.

Key Alignment:

~ From Trikonasana or Parsvakonasana, with your top hand on your hip, step your back leg forward and place your lower hand about 6–10 inches in front of your foot, to the pinky-toe side.

~ Spread your toes and lift your back leg up. Keep the bottom leg strong and extend from your tailbone energetically down your standing leg, anchoring firmly into the Earth.

~ Lift from your back inner thigh, being sure not to take your leg behind you; keep it in line with your body or slightly forward so you can look down your body and see your back foot if you wanted.

~ From the inside, turn your belly and heart upwards, drawing the shoulders onto your back and reaching your top hand to the sky.

~ Extend out from your pelvis in all directions like a star!

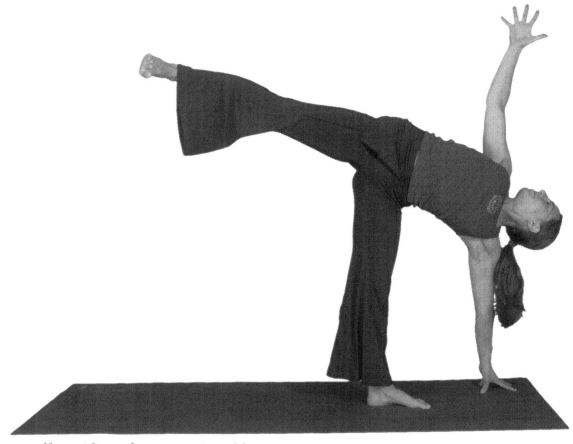

Ardha Chandrasana (Half Moon Pose)

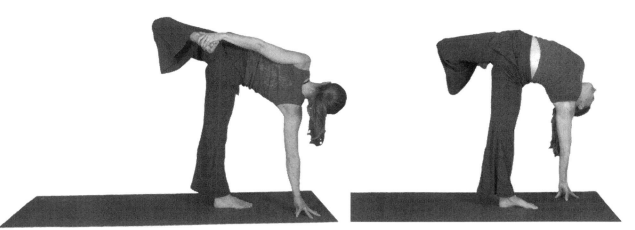

Ardha Chandra Chapasana (Sugar Cane Half Moon)

HANUMANASANA (SPLITS)
ARDHA HANUMANASANA (HALF HANUMAN OR RUNNER'S LUNGE)

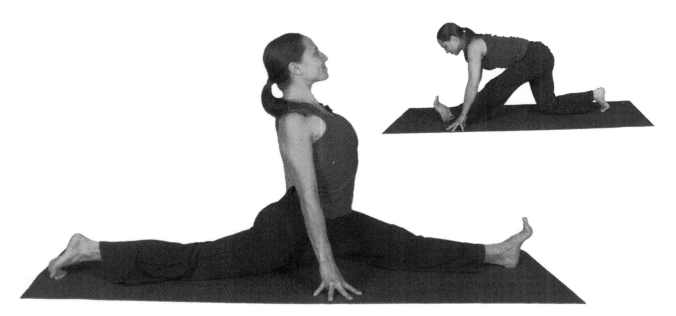

Significance: Taking a great leap. Deep opening. Devotion. Boldness. Vitality.

Benefits: Creates strength and balance. Stretches the legs and hips deeply, including the hip flexors and hamstrings. Stimulates internal organs and functions.

Cautions/Modifications: Modify with Runner's Lunge, which is also a good prep pose for Hanumanasana. Go only as far as your body is ready, in alignment. Use blocks to support your hands if you'd like. Do not force this if you have hamstring or groin injuries. However, if you can do this pose with optimal alignment, it can actually be therapeutic for those injuries.

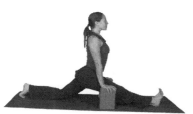

Key Alignment:

- Start in Runner's Lunge, with one foot forward and your back knee down.

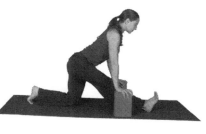

- Take a deep breath, spread your toes and hug your muscles to the bones.

- Draw your legs toward each other, creating integration and safety.

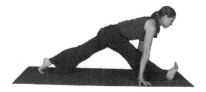

- Widen the inner thighs back and apart, then, keeping that, scoop your tailbone firmly toward the front foot.
- Extend from the pelvis outward, going deeper into the pose.
- Repeat: Integrate, Align, Extend. Breath by breath go deeper.
- Keep your front foot and knee pointed up, your back foot and knee pointed down.
- Once in the pose there are many variations. Start with these two: (1) Lift your torso upwards and curl back slightly as you extend through your legs to get a deeper hip flexor stretch. (2) Bend forward over your front leg.

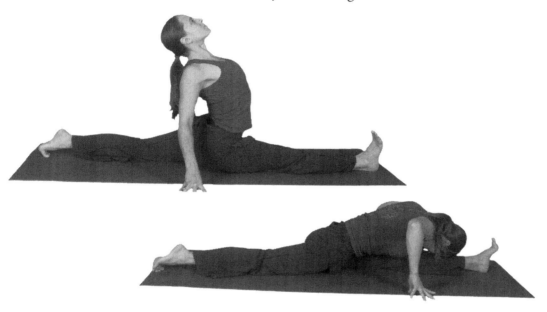

Transition through Down Dog on fingertips

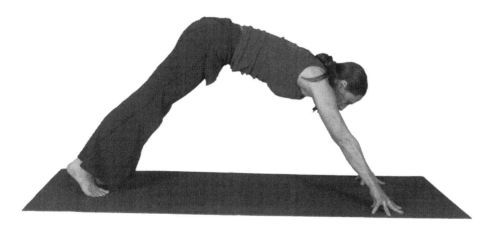

Eka Pada Rajakapotasana prep (Pigeon)

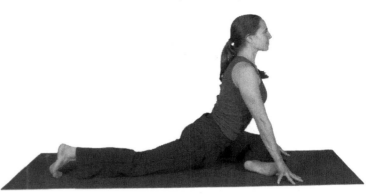

Significance: Spaciousness. Receptivity. Compassion. Modesty. Reverence.

Benefits: Stretches the hips, groin, and other areas depending on the variation. Stimulates internal organs. Can be an excellent release to move stuck energy in the hips.

Cautions/Modifications: If you have knee, ankle, or hip conditions, you will likely want to modify in Thread The Needle. If your hips are tight, keep your front foot near your pelvis and point your toes back in line with your shin to make the pose more accessible and easier on your knees. There should be NO pain in your knees here. If there is, modify. Check the angle of your foot to be sure it's not turning in or out compared to your shin. You may need to do a thigh stretch before doing this pose in order to open up your hips and have less tension on the knees.

Key Alignment:

- From Downward Dog, step one foot forward and towards the opposite wrist.
- Spread your toes and keep the ankle aligned. Take your knee out to the side, near the edge of your mat.

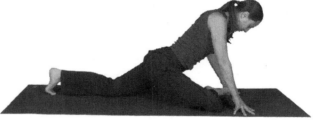

- With your back toes tucked under, step your leg further back. With your hands or fingertips on the floor in front of your leg, take a deep breath.

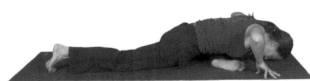

- Integrate, drawing your legs toward each other, widening the back thigh and squaring your pelvis forward.
- Draw the front hip downward even as you continue to spin the inner thigh back on the leg that is behind you.
- Be sure your back shin stays strong and the heel doesn't roll out.
- Lengthen forward with your breath, coming to your forearms as you're ready.
- From your pelvis, extend in all directions. Play with the integration, refinement, and extension as you breathe deeply into your hips.

Thread the Needle is a non-weight bearing variation of Pigeon

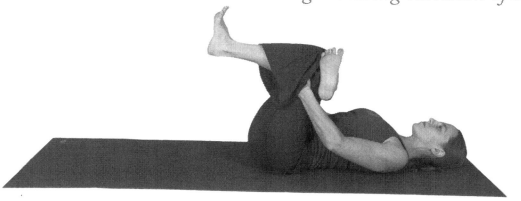

Eka Pada Rajakapotasana variation (Pigeon Thigh Stretch)
Eka Pada Bhekasana (Thigh Stretch on Belly)

Significance: Joyful. Capable. Generous. Shining from the inside. Willingness to serve.

Benefits: Stretches the hips, thighs, chest, shoulders and abdomen. Strengthens and improves balance. Stimulates internal organs and circulation.

Cautions/Modifications: If you have a knee injury, stretching your thighs and hips is very important,

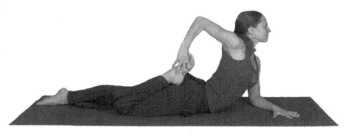

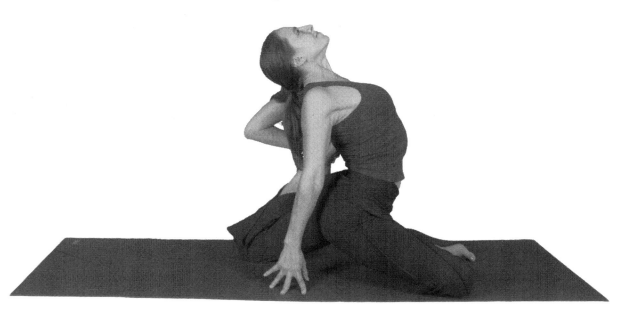

but be sure to do it in a way that is optimally aligned and in a variation that works for your body. If there is cartilage damage, you can put a rolled up washcloth or small towel behind your knee to create space. Don't force: you do not want to increase the injury, but heal instead. Modify with a thigh stretch on your belly or side. Warm up by stretching the hamstrings and hips, calves and hip flexors in other poses first. A very important aspect of the alignment that many beginners don't get at first in this pose is the extension of stretching out. It is strong, and when done after you have integrated, creates space in the knee joint for more circulation.

Pigeon Thigh Stretch

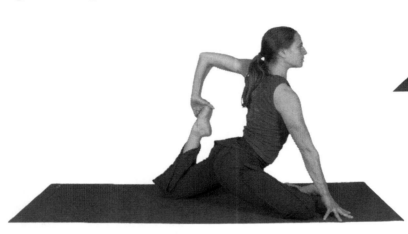

Key Alignment:

~ From pigeon prep, with one leg bent in front and one leg behind, take a deep breath and allow a spaciousness inside.

~ Integrate, make your legs strong and draw them towards each other, squaring your hips.

~ Widen the inner thighs, especially the back inner thigh without letting the back shin or heel roll out.

~ Reach your tailbone firmly down and forward as the front hip draws down.

~ Bend your back knee and take the top of the back foot with the same side hand.

~ Press your foot and hand into each other, extending brightly from the pelvis out through both legs. For a deeper stretch, spin your elbow toward the sky and take the heel toward the outer hip.

~ The front hand can be on the floor, on a block, on your thigh, up in the air, or behind you on the mat.

~ Reintegrate, refine, and extend, lifting your torso upwards as your tailbone reaches forward.

~Let your chest open as your shoulders draw back, heart bright!

~ Breathe, and clear any tension with your breath.

Setu Bandha Sarvangasana (Bridge pose)

Significance: Open-heartedness. Vulnerability without weakness. Adaptability. Bridging one world and another. Rooted in acceptance.

Benefits: Calming and revitalizing. Stimulates the organs, immune system and hormones. Stretches the hip flexors, chest, shoulders and spine. Strengthens and rejuvenates the legs. Relieves stress, anxiety, depression, fatigue, headache, insomnia, and back pain.

Cautions/Modifications: If you have a blood pressure condition, transition slowly out of this pose, giving yourself time to regulate. If you have neck injury, be sure that you can perform this in alignment or do so only with a teacher. It is crucial that NO vertebrae are on the floor, and that you keep your head neutral. Pressing back through your head from the ears, and back through your shoulders as well, will create a lift in the cervical spine and take the vertebrae off the ground. If you have a hip injury, hold a block between your inner thighs and spin them down while reaching your tailbone up. Also, holding a block between your shins can be very helpful while learning optimal alignment in this pose.

Key Alignment:

- Lie on your back and place your feet beneath your knees, slightly narrower than hip-width apart. Feet are parallel.

- With an inhale, lengthen your torso. Then, press your elbows and head gently back, lift your heart and draw your shoulder blades more fully onto your back, shoulders back and toward your spine.

- Inhale and lift your hips. Spread your toes to keep your legs strong, shins steady.

- If you're able, interlace your hands beneath you. Otherwise, take your hands outward bending your elbows, so you can get your shoulders back more fully.

- Lean from one side to the other and take the shoulders under you, heads of the arm bones pressing back into the Earth.

- Press from your upper palate (roof of your mouth) back through your head.

- Lift your heart higher, groins back, tailbone scooped up.

- Extend your head back into the Earth, and also stretch out through your throat, heart, hips, leg bones, and all four corners of your feet.

- When you are ready to come down, lower your hips first so you keep the natural curve of your spine. Rest for a few breaths before repeating or moving on in your practice.

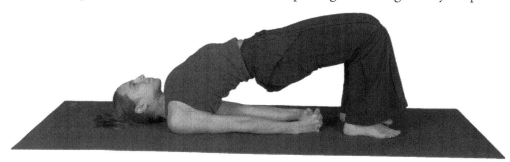

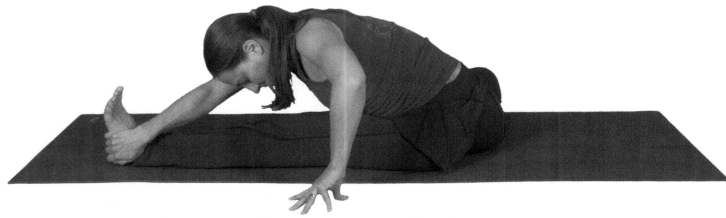

Janu Sirsasana (Head to Knee Pose)

Significance: Patience. Gratitude. Deepening. Tolerance. Kindness.

Benefits: Calming, grounding. Stretches the hips, hamstrings, groins, spine, and back, particularly the lower sides of your back. Stimulates the internal organs, improving digestion. Helps relieve stress, anxiety, fatigue, high blood pressure, insomnia, and headache.

Cautions/Modifications: Don't think of this as head to knee pose—that's just how the Sanskrit translates. Maybe think heart to knee, or head to shin. Regardless, don't lead with your head or you'll tend to round the lower back and harden the upper back. If you have knee injuries, straighten both legs out in a straddle position for Parsva Upavistha Konasana. If your lower back rounds when you sit or you have a back injury, sit up on one or more blankets. If you're pregnant, don't bend as far forward.

Key Alignment:

- Sit with one leg straight and one bent, knee out, foot towards the groin, thighs wide—separated at least 90-degrees—so your hips are facing diagonally between the two.

- Spread your toes, make your muscles hug the bones, and send your inner thighs into the ground. You can also manually spin the thighs back, using your hands to widen your sit bones, hamstrings, femurs, and groins.

- Anchor your thighbones and tailbone down.

- Inhale to lengthen your torso, then turn toward the straight leg and fold forward as you exhale.

- Use the hand that is on your straight leg side to press into the ground beside you and help lengthen your torso. Take the opposite hand across to the outer calf, pressing hand and shin into each other. You may also reach your hand to the foot if you're able.

- Use your breath to twist deeper, keeping your lower back long and lifted.

- Extend from your pelvis through your feet and spine. Breathe. Be sure to move on your inhale when you are ready to come out of the pose.

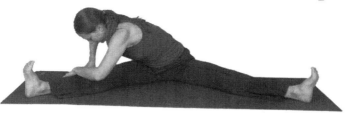

Parsva Upavistha Konasana

Supta Padangusthasana variation (Hamstring Hug)

Significance: Grounded. Safe. Supported. Integrated. Self-honoring.

Benefits: Balances and clears the hips and back. Roots the femurs. Stretches hips and hamstrings. Helpful for lowering high blood pressure, improving digestion, stimulating hormones and internal organs, and relieving back and hip pain. Can also help hamstring strains.

Cautions/Modifications: If you have a hamstring strain, place your hands behind that spot as you do this pose. If you are unable to comfortably take your hands behind your leg, use a strap. If your hamstrings are very tight, keep your top knee bent.

Key Alignment:

- Lying on your back, take your legs together and spread your toes to tone the legs.

- Press your inner thighs into the Earth, then scoop your tail bone toward your heels.

- Inhale and lift one leg up, interlacing your hands behind your thigh. Keep your hands, wrists, and arms integrated, shoulders drawing back. Head is neutral, with space beneath your neck.

- Press your top thigh into your hands, your lower inner thigh into the Earth.

- Extend from your pelvis through your feet, especially the heels.

- The point of this pose is to get the femurs *back (as in towards the back plane of your body).* This roots them more deeply in your hips and helps balance and heal your back and hips.

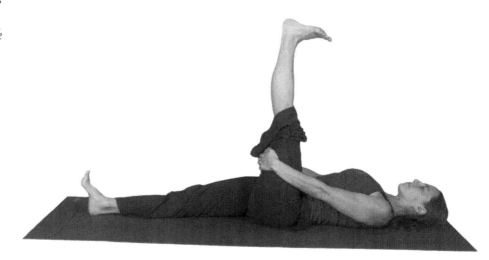

SUPINE TWIST
(FINISHING TWIST/ROTATOR CUFF AND SHOULDER STRENGTHENER)

Significance: Neutralizing. Cleansing. Freeing. Soothing. Nurturing.

Benefits: Calming, clearing. Strengthens shoulders and back. Stretches spine, hips, and chest. Stimulates, detoxes, and cleanses internal organs.

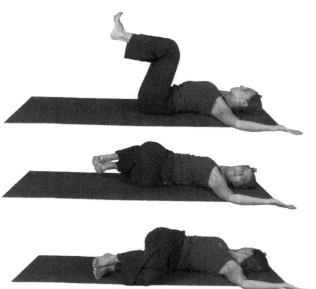

Cautions/Modifications: This pose can be used as a finishing twist, or therapeutically to strengthen the rotator cuffs. The difference is with the first you hold to one side for several breaths, and with the strengthener you go from side to side with each breath. As with all but the most gentle twists, avoid during pregnancy. Be sure to keep the shoulders back the whole time.

Key Alignment:

~ Lying on your back, take a breath to lengthen your spine and press your shoulders back.

~ Inhale to lift your legs—knees close together; toes spread—keep strength and awareness in your legs and stability in your pelvis.

~ Keeping your head gently back and the heads of your arm bones firmly rooted back, inhale again.

~ Exhale, and take your legs to one side.

~ If this is a finishing twist for you, take several breaths here, turning your head to the opposite side if you'd like. Breathe up and down your spine, and into your organs and hips. When ready, inhale to neutral, exhale to the other side.

~ If you are using this as a rotator cuff strengthener, inhale to center and exhale to the other side, repeating side to side with your breath. Head stays neutral in this exercise. Pin the heads of the arm bones back firmly and don't let them lift up—this is what strengthens the stabilizing muscles in your shoulders.

~ Inhale back to center.

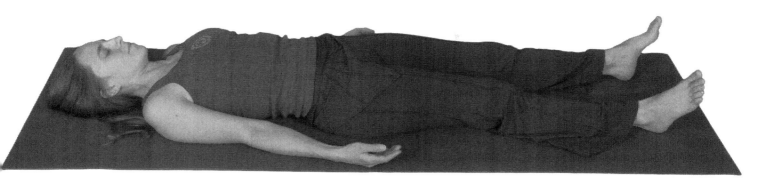

Savasana (Corpse Pose—pronounced "shavasana")

Significance: Completeness. Death as rebirth. Total surrender. Mindfulness. Transition.

Benefits: Calming. Relaxing. Integrates the benefits of the practice on every level. Allows the fluids of your body to distribute evenly. Reduces fatigue, headache, insomnia. Helpful to lower blood pressure and the heart rate.

Cautions/Modifications: If you have respiratory troubles, or are pregnant, you can recline with your chest and head lifted on a bolster. You can also lie on your left side if you're pregnant. If you are uncomfortable in Savasana, and have aligned as optimally as you can, try using a strap or sandbags to stabilize your shins and thighs parallel to each other. If you have an injury you may need to maintain a degree of effort to stay optimally aligned. For instance, if your SI (sacroiliac) ligaments are loose, you may need to keep that area slightly toned and not let your legs roll out. Avoid putting something under your knees or head if possible, as this flattens the natural curves of the spine. You can roll something small under your neck if you need support. If you are experiencing fear or anxiety, try placing your hands on your belly, or even rolling onto your belly, placing your head on your hands, and doing downward facing Savasana.

Key Alignment:

- Lie on your back. Be sure you are comfortable, and cover up with a blanket if possible.

- Take a deep breath and soften.

- Do all of the alignment to set yourself up optimally: legs parallel, shins drawing inward, thighs back, tailbone toward your knees, long upper body, shoulders back.

- Then, with your next breath, relax as fully as you can. Allow your arms and legs to be at a comfortable angle and do what they will, rolling out or in.

- Soften, releasing your entire weight to the Earth. Let your thighs be heavy, your ribs rest back. Even your internal organs and eyes can sink back.

- Maintain your focus on your breath, allowing it full freedom as you integrate and rest.

Modifications and Optional Poses

Nearly anything can be modified. Anytime a pose doesn't work for your body, for any reason, you can substitute something different that does.

In the key poses section you will see modifications offered for poses to give you ideas. If a modification isn't included here on a pose you need to adapt, use your own discernment and get creative. On that note, if there are any poses you are unsure about or know are not right for you, modify or skip them. Tailor these practices to your own unique needs.

Also included in the sequences are *Optional* poses, which are intended for you to do only if you already have experience with them and feel confident doing them on your own.

A Note to Female Riders:

It is important to note that a yoga practice changes depending on many things such as energy, health, the time of year, or the time of month. One of the considerations in the approach to a yoga practice is a woman's menstrual cycle. Every woman is different, but in general menstruation is a time to tone things back and rest.

During your cycle keep in mind these three things:

1. **Honor the life force.** There is a fundamental force of energy present during the menstrual cycle. It is a process to be nurtured and respected. When the energy of this time is disrespected, the flow can be disrupted which could lead to health problems and premature aging, so it is crucial to know what your body needs during menstruation and allow yourself to rest. Honor the life force. It is a powerful time. Sometimes it is good to take a day off from asana, and it's a perfect time to incorporate more restorative practices. Every woman is different, so use your intuition and see what your body's needs are during this time.

2. **Avoid Inversions.** The menstrual cycle naturally flows downward. Let it. Turning upside down goes against the natural flow and can cause disruption or even stop the flow of menstruation. Once the cycle is *completely* finished, however, it is recommended to immediately incorporate inversions and poses that tone the reproductive organs. This helps to create balance.

3. **Don't over contract.** As with avoiding inversions, you want to keep the flow of Prana headed downward. If you overly contract your belly or abdominals the energy gets pulled up. It is wise to back off on the amount of toning and core conditioning you do at this time.

If you'd like to learn more about yoga specific to women or learn what poses to apply for different conditions women experience, Geeta Iyengar's writing is an excellent place to start.

Practice Sequences

These practices offer a wide range of possibilities. Think of the following section as a "Choose Your Own Adventure." Roll out your mat, greet your Dragon, and go for a ride.

Your practice may look different than this. You don't necessarily need to use all of these practices or poses. Do what is best for your body and your life.

The practices are as follows:

Awaken the Dragon: Flow, power, movement prep, and key poses

Spaciousness and Strength: Standing poses and balances, plus essential poses

Balance and Bravery: Standing balances and arm balances

Splendor of the Heart: Chest openers and backbends

Deeper Insight: Hip openers

Purity and Flow: Twists and connections

Waves of Pulsation: Forward bends and optional inversions

Cradle of Healing: Restorative bliss and deep healing

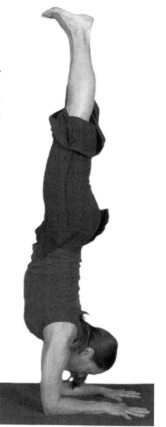

Pincha Mayurasana
(Peacock feather Pose)

Here's how these practices are presented for you, clearly defined with purpose and focus:

The Virtues are the qualities you cultivate, contemplate, and embody as you do the practice.

The Focus is the general postural theme.

The Apex is the pose (or poses) that serve as the zenith of the practice. They generally are the most challenging or most in-depth asanas in the sequence.

When you see this symbol **>** it means you can do one pose right after the other on the same side. For example, Warrior II > Goddess Warrior > Triangle Pose means you go into Goddess Warrior from Warrior II, and then proceed right into Triangle on the same side. After finishing that flow, you can transition through Down Dog or a Vinyasa to repeat on the other side.

The Dance of Intention: Awaken the Dragon

The Virtues: Interconnection, Grace, and Balance of Love, Wisdom and Power in each moment.

The Focus: Flow and Power

The Apex: Flying Warrior

This practice can serve as a stand-alone practice or a mindful movement prep. It is also a great way to start your day. Let your intention be reflected in each pose.

SEQUENCE:

Tadasana—spread your wings and breathe

Uttanasana—pulse with your breath

Rotator Cuff Twist

Scorpion Twist

Down Dog (pulse, bending one knee at a time with breath)

Plank (optional: inchworm with push-up, or do plank with one leg lifted)

Chaturanga

Cobra

Down Dog

Pulsing Parsvottanasana variation (3 breaths x 3 on each side)

Uttanasana to standing

Twisting Lunges

Flying Warrior

Optional transition point-

Anjaneyasana

Runner's Lunge

Vinyasa

Vira II > Goddess Warrior > Trikonasana

Vinyasa

Pigeon Thigh Stretch

Pigeon

Uttanasana

Janu Sirsasana

Hamstring Hug

Twist

Meditation or Savasana

124

Optional transition point means that from Flying Warrior you could go into any other type of activity feeling warmed up for stable, powerful movement. You could insert your workout or run/bike/hike and so on; then return to yoga and continue from the transition point with the rest of the practice serving as a cool down and mindful stretch.

This is a wonderful practice to do before adventures of any kind.

This is also a good way to go for a short ride on the wings of Shakti, get your blood flowing, and connect your intention to the manifest world through breath and movement.

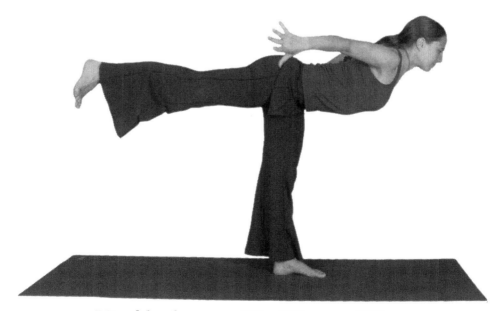

Virabhadrasana III (Warrior III)

125

Awaken the Dragon

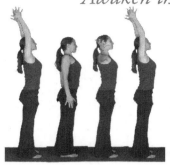

Tadasana
spread your wings

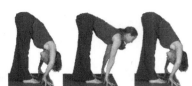

Uttanasana
pulse with your breath

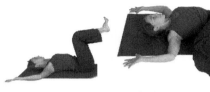

Rotator Cuff Twist - Inhale center, Exhale to twist
go from side to side with your breath
press your shoulders firmly back

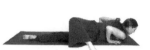 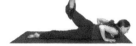

Scorpion twist from side to side

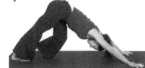

Down Dog, bend knees
pulse with your breath

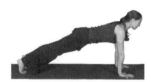

Plank, hold 3 breaths
Optional: push-ups or one leg push-ups

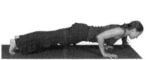

Chaturanga
lower to belly

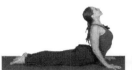

Bhujangasana
Cobra Pose

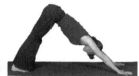

Down Dog
enjoy your breath

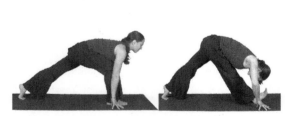

Pulse from lunge to straight leg stretch
3 breaths straight, 1 breath bent knee
3 times each side

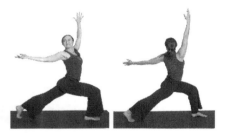

Twisting lunges with straight back leg
side to side 5 to 10 times each side

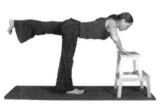

Optional variation for
Vira III with chair

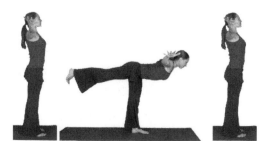

Flying Warrior III
pulse Tadasana to Vira III to Tadasana
5 to 10 times each side

* OPTIONAL
TRANSITION
POINT

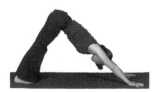

Down Dog
enjoy your breath

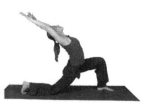

Anjaneyasana
both sides

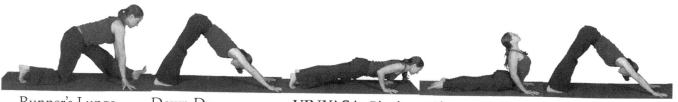

Runner's Lunge
both sides

Down Dog
enjoy your breath

VINYASA: Plank > Chaturanga > Cobra > Down Dog

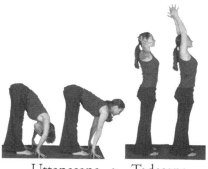

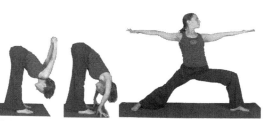

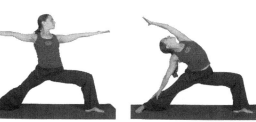

Uttanasana > Tadasana

Uttanasana
shoulder stretch

FLOW: Warrior II > Goddess Warrior >

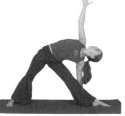

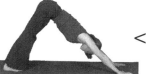

< VINYASA >

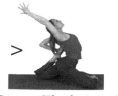

Trikonasana > Down Dog
repeat FLOW on other side

Pigeon Thigh Stretch
both sides

Pigeon Forward Fold
both sides

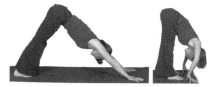

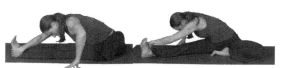

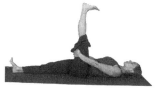

Down Dog > Uttanasana

Janu Sirsasana on both sides

Hamstring Hug
both sides

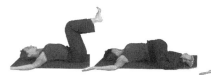

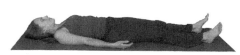

Finishing Twist
go to one side and take 3 to 5 deep breaths
then inhale through center to the other side

Savasana
relax for several minutes
enjoy your breath

Spaciousness and Strength

The Virtues: Grounded Strength and Steadiness, in complete balance with Spacious Sensitivity.

The Focus: Standing poses and essential postures for whole body benefit.

The Apex: Ardha Chandrasana and variations

SEQUENCE:

Tadasana, lift and lower arms with breath

Uttanasana, extend and bow with breath

Lunge Twist

Down Dog

Lunge Twist (other side)

Uttanasana

Tadasana

Goddess Crescent (Crescent Lunge with backbend, optional)

Uttanasana shoulder stretch

Surya Namaskar with Crescent > Vira III

Vinyasa with Vira II to Goddess Warrior

Vinyasa

Garudasana

Parsvottanasana

Parsvakonasana > Trikonasana > Ardha Chandrasana

Parivrtta Parsvakonasana (bound optional)

Vinyasa

Trikonasana > Ardha Chandrasana > Ardha Chandra Chapasana (optional) > Parivrtta Ardha Chandrasana (optional) > Vira I

Prasarita Padottanasana (with headstand optional)

Vinyasa

Uttanasana

Vrksasana (Tree Pose)

Vinyasa

Pigeon Thigh Stretch

Pigeon

Uttanasana

Parsvottanasana > Parivrtta Trikonasana

Uttanasana

Janu Sirsasana

Ardha Matsyendrasana

Setu Bandha Sarvangasana

Supta Padangusthasana (Hamstring Hug)

Parivrtta Supta Padangusthasana (or any finishing twist)

Savasana

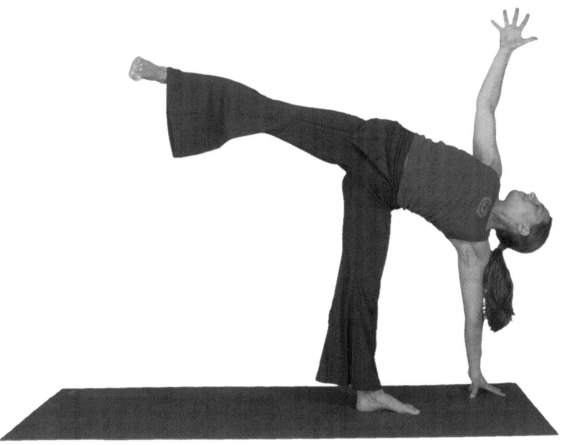

Ardha Chandrasana (Half Moon Pose)

Spaciousness and Strength

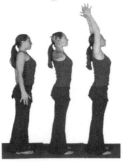
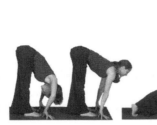
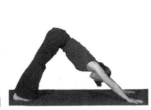

Tadasana
spread your wings

Uttanasana
pulse with your breath

Lunge Twist on each side
pause in Down Dog in between and breathe

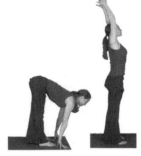
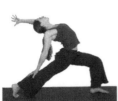
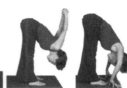
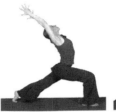

Uttanasana to
Tadasana

Goddess
Crescent

Uttanasana
shoulder stretch

FLOW: Crescent Lunge > Vira III
transition back to Crescent Lunge

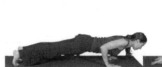
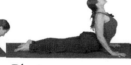
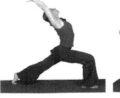

Chaturanga
lower to belly

Bhujangasana
Cobra pose

Down Dog
enjoy your breath

FLOW: Other side

< VINYASA >

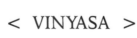
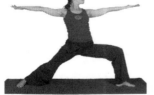

< VINYASA >

FLOW: Warrior II > Goddesss Warrior
repeat FLOW on other side

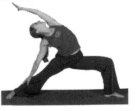
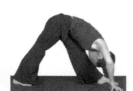
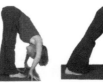
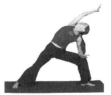
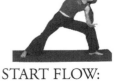

Garudasana (Eagle Pose)
both sides

Parsvottanasana
both sides

Pause. Breathe. Feel.

START FLOW:
High Parsvakonasana >

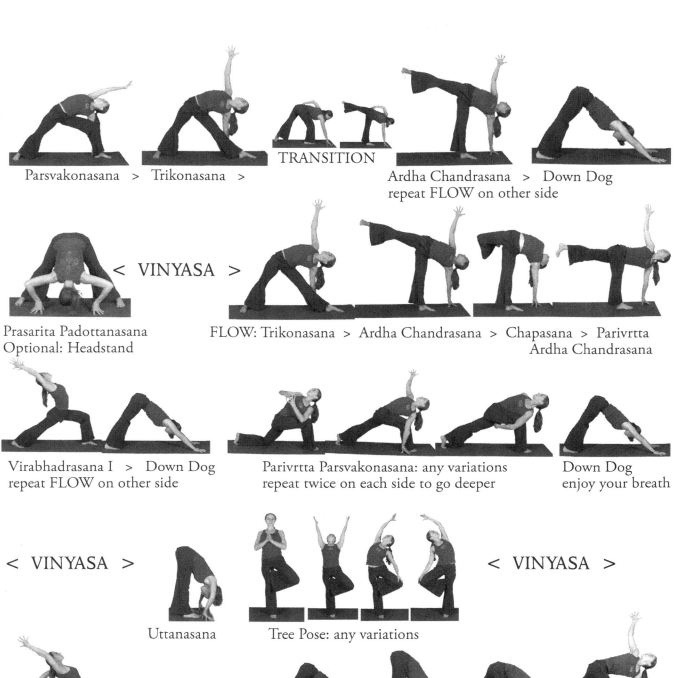

Parsvakonasana > Trikonasana > TRANSITION Ardha Chandrasana > Down Dog
repeat FLOW on other side

Prasarita Padottanasana
Optional: Headstand

< VINYASA >

FLOW: Trikonasana > Ardha Chandrasana > Chapasana > Parivrtta
Ardha Chandrasana

Virabhadrasana I > Down Dog
repeat FLOW on other side

Parivrtta Parsvakonasana: any variations
repeat twice on each side to go deeper

Down Dog
enjoy your breath

< VINYASA >

Uttanasana

Tree Pose: any variations

< VINYASA >

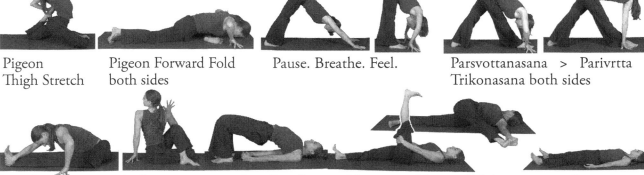

Pigeon
Thigh Stretch

Pigeon Forward Fold
both sides

Pause. Breathe. Feel.

Parsvottanasana > Parivrtta
Trikonasana both sides

Janu Sirsasana
both sides

Ardha
Matsyendrasana

Setu Bandha
Sarvangasana

Hamstring Hug and Twist

Savasana

Balance and Bravery

The Virtues: Willingness and Awareness, balanced with Skillful Courage.

The Focus: Standing balances and arm balances

The Apex: Natarajasana, Parivrtta Hasta Padangusthasana, Urdhva Vrksasana, Pincha Mayurasana

SEQUENCE:

Balasana

Adho Mukha Svanasana

Vinyasa to Lunge Twist

Vinyasa to Crescent to Vira III

Vinyasa to Tadasana

Garudasana

Uttanasana shoulder stretch

Vira II > Parsvakonasana > Trikonasana > Ardha Chandrasana

Vinyasa to Anjaneyasana

Urdhva Vrksasana (Handstand optional)

Pincha Mayurasana (Forearm Stand optional)

Runner's Lunge

Vinyasa to Anjaneyasana thigh stretch

Vinyasa

Parsvottanasana

Utthita Hasta Padangusthasana

Parivrtta Hasta Padangusthasana

Vinyasa with Shalabhasana

Vashisthasana > Wild Thing

Down Dog to standing

Baby Natarajasana

Bakasana (Crow Pose, with any other arm balance variations you'd like to do)

Vinyasa

Balasana

Adho Mukha Svanasana

Pigeon

Uttanasana

Janu Sirsasana

Ardha Matsyendrasana

Upavistha Konsasana

Baddha Konasana

Supta Padangusthasana

Twist

Savasana

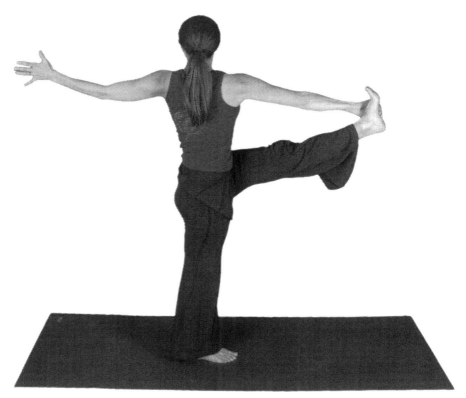

Parivrtta Hasta Padangusthasana
(Revolved Hand to Big Toe Pose)

Balance and Bravery

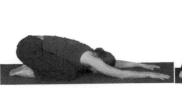

Balasana: Child's Pose
breathe into your body

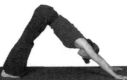

Down Dog
move as you like

< VINYASA >

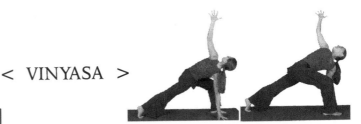

Lunge Twist on each side
transition through Down Dog

< VINYASA >

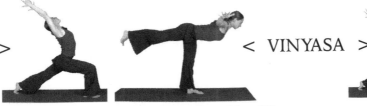

FLOW: Crescent Lunge (Vira I) > Vira III
transition back to Crescent Lunge

< VINYASA >

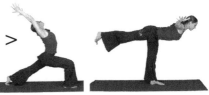

FLOW: Other side

< VINYASA >

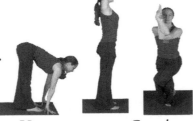

Uttanasana to
Tadasana

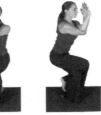

Garudasana (Eagle Pose)
both sides

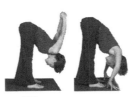

Uttanasana
shoulder stretch

< VINYASA >

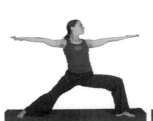

FLOW: Vira II > Parsvakonasana > Trikonasana > Ardha Chandrasana
repeat FLOW on other side

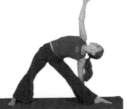

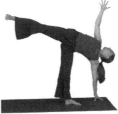

< VINYASA >

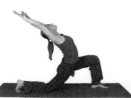

Anjaneyasana
both sides

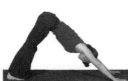

Down Dog
enjoy your breath

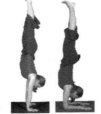

Optional:
Handstand and/or
Pincha Mayurasana

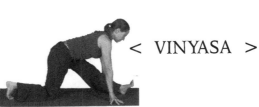

Ardha Hanumanasana
Runner's Lunge

< VINYASA >

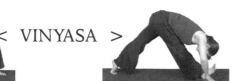 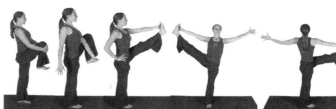 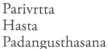

< VINYASA >

Anjaneyasana
Thigh Stretch

Parsvottanasana
variation

Uthitta Hasta Padangusthasana
any variation, both sides

Parivrtta
Hasta
Padangusthasana

< VINYASA >

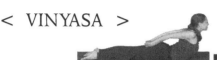 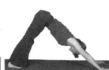 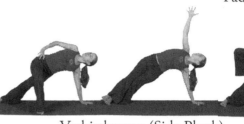

Shalabhasana
(Locust Pose)

Down Dog
enjoy your breath

Vashisthasana (Side Plank)
any variation, into Wild Thing

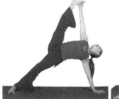 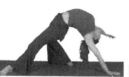 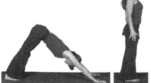 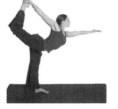

Vashisthasana > Wild Thing

Down Dog > Tadasana

Baby Natarajasana
(Dancer's Pose)

Bakasana
(Crow Pose)
and other balances

< VINYASA >

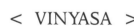 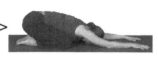 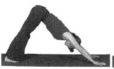 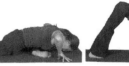

Balasana: Child's Pose
enjoy your breath

Pigeon Forward Fold
both sides

  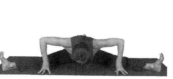 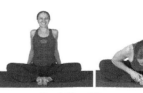

Janu Sirsasana

Ardha
Matsyendrasana

Upavistha Konasana

Baddha Konasana

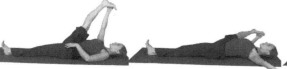 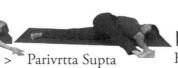 

Supta Padangusthasana: any variations > Parivrtta Supta
Padangusthasana

Hug and Rock

Savasana

Splendor of the Heart

The Virtues: Service and Devotion bringing Illumination, Awakening and Freedom

The Focus: Chest openers and backbends

The Apex: Urdhva Dhanurasana and variations

SEQUENCE:

Adho Mukha Svanasana (Down Dog)

Plank > Chaturanga > floor

Cobra

Adho Mukha Svanasana

Straight leg lunge with twist (pausing first in the lunge before twisting) (both sides)

Adho Mukha Svanasana

Plank—hold (optional push-ups)

Chaturanga—hold > floor

Cobra

Adho Mukha Svanasana

Anjaneyasana (both sides)

Uttanasana

Tadasana (pause, breathe, feel)

Uttanasana with hands interlaced behind for shoulder stretch

Parivrtta Parsvakonasana (back heel lifted, both sides)

Vinyasa with cobra, hold Chaturanga

Trikonasana with back bend > Parsvakonasana with arm inside leg (both sides)

Vinyasa

Trikonasana > Ardha Chandrasana > Ardha Chandra Chapasana (both sides)

Adho Mukha Svanasana

Standing baby cradle (or pigeon)

Tuck and Pike hop ups > Handstand prep from Down dog

Urdhva Vrksasana (Handstand)

Pincha Mayurasana (optional)

Adho Mukha Svanasana

Pigeon Thigh Stretch

Supta Virasana (coming out through modified Kapotasana optional)

Adho Mukha Svanasana

Urdhva Dhanurasana (repeat)

Eka Pada Urdhva Dhanurasana (optional)

Drop backs if you're feelin' it

Adho Mukha Svanasana

Uttanasana

Parsva Uttanasana

Parsvottanasana

Parivrtta Trikonasana

Uttanasana

Janu Sirsasana

Ardha Matsyendrasana

Ardha Baddha Padma Paschimottanasana to Ardha Matsyendrasana II

Supta Padangusthasana

Parivrtta Supta Padangusthasana

Supta Balasana or Supta Tadasana

Savasana

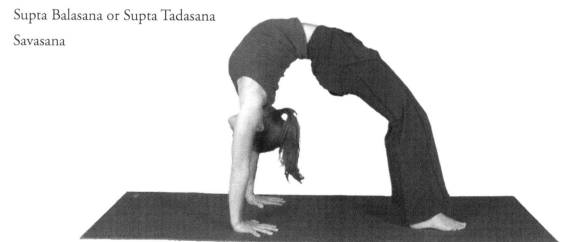

Urdhva Dhanurasana (Upward Facing Bow Pose)   137

Splendor of the Heart

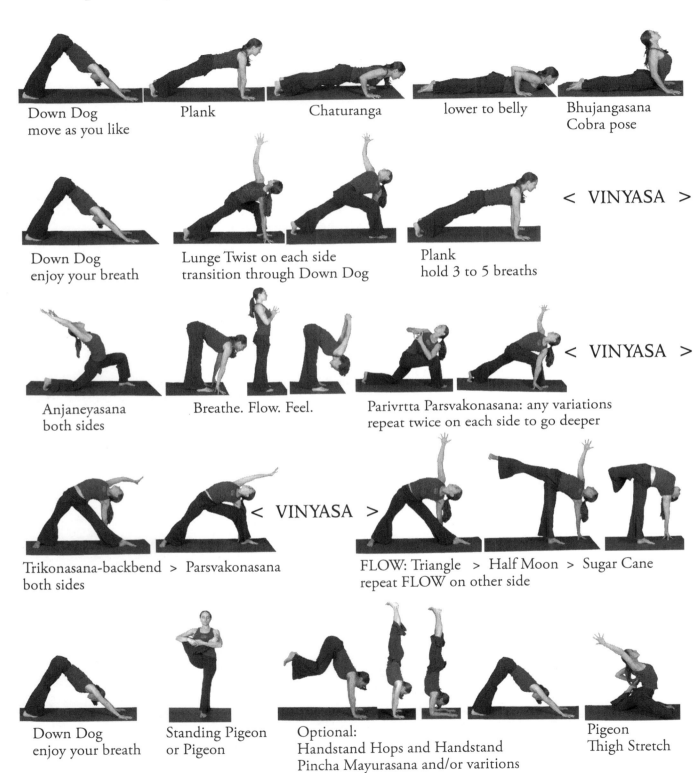

Down Dog
move as you like

Plank

Chaturanga

lower to belly

Bhujangasana
Cobra pose

< VINYASA >

Down Dog
enjoy your breath

Lunge Twist on each side
transition through Down Dog

Plank
hold 3 to 5 breaths

< VINYASA >

Anjaneyasana
both sides

Breathe. Flow. Feel.

Parivrtta Parsvakonasana: any variations
repeat twice on each side to go deeper

< VINYASA >

Trikonasana-backbend > Parsvakonasana
both sides

FLOW: Triangle > Half Moon > Sugar Cane
repeat FLOW on other side

Down Dog
enjoy your breath

Standing Pigeon
or Pigeon

Optional:
Handstand Hops and Handstand
Pincha Mayurasana and/or varitions

Pigeon
Thigh Stretch

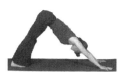
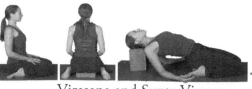
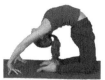

Down Dog
enjoy your breath

Virasana and Supta Virasana: any variation
(Hero's Pose and Reclining Hero)

Optional:
Kapotasana
transition

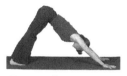
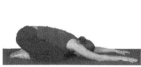
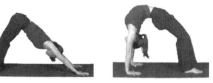
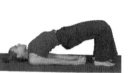

Down Dog
enjoy your breath

Child's Pose

Urdhva Dhanurasana
(repeat)

or Setu Bandha
Sarvangasana

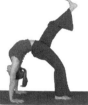
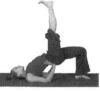

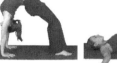

Eka Pada
Urdhva
Dhanurasana

or Eka Pada
Setu Bandha
Sarvangasana

Drop Backs if you're feelin' it

Windshield Wipers
slow, with your breath

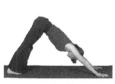
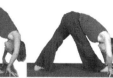

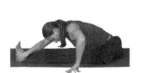

Pause. Feel. Breathe.

Parsvottanasana > Parivrtta
Trikonasana: both sides

Parsva Uttanasana

Janu Sirsasana

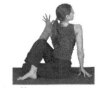
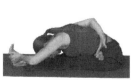
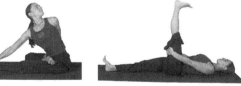

Ardha
Matsyendrasana

Ardha Baddha Padma Paschimottanasana
into Ardha Matsyendrasana II (or variations)

Supta Padangusthasana

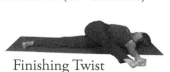

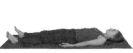

Finishing Twist

Hug and Rock

Savasana

Deeper Insight

The Virtues: Self-Study, Wisdom, and Humility as they bring Insight and Revelation

The Focus: Hip openers

The Apex: Vishvamitrasana, Krounchasana, Surya Yantrasana, Parivrtta Janu Sirsasana

SEQUENCE:

Adho Mukha Savasana (lie on your belly with your hands under your head and breathe)

Balasana

Down dog

Uttanasana

Tadasana, pulse with breath

Wide Uttanasana with shoulder stretch

Dragon Lunge with twist

Vinyasa

Parsvottanasana

Vinyasa

Anjaneyasana

Down dog

Parsvakonasana > Trikonasana > Ardha Chandrasana

Pigeon with twist

Vinyasa

Pigeon thigh stretch

Runner's Lunge

Hanumanasana

Lunge with shoulder behind shin > Vishvamitrasana (optional)

Vinyasa with Shalabhasana

Uttanasana

Janu Sirsasana

Triang Mukhaipada Paschimottanasana (optional)

Krounchasana (Heron Pose - optional)

Surya Yantrasana (Sundial Pose - optional)

Parsva Upavistha Konasana

Upavistha Konasana

Parivrtta Janu Sirsasana (x2)

Supine Pigeon

Ardha happy baby

Finishing Twist

Savasana

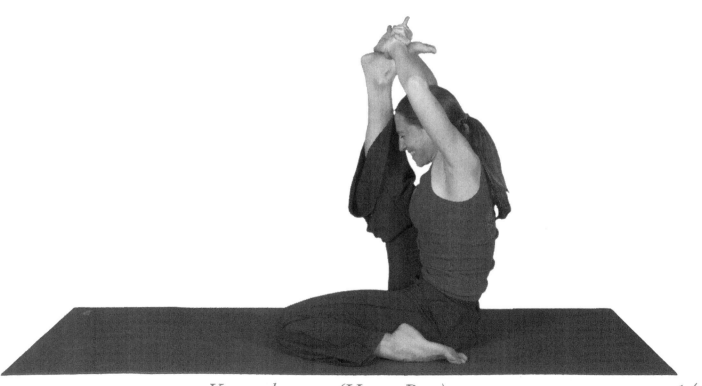

Krounchasana (Heron Pose)

Deeper Insight

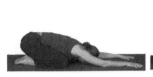 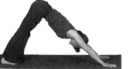 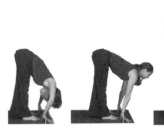 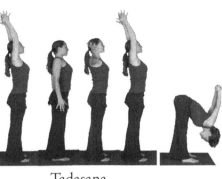

Balasana: Child's Pose
breathe into your body

Down Dog
move as you like

Uttanasana
pulse with your breath

Tadasana
spread your wings

< VINYASA >   < VINYASA >

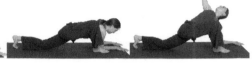 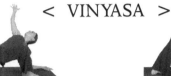

Dragon Lunge Twist
both sides

Parsvottanasana
both sides

< VINYASA >

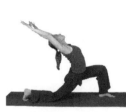 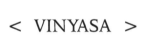 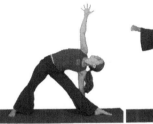

Anjaneyasana
both sides

FLOW: Parsvakonasana > Trikonasana > Ardha Chandrasana
repeat FLOW on other side

< VINYASA >

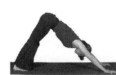 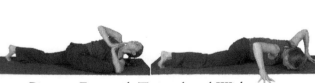 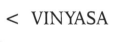

Breathe. Feel.

Pigeon: Forward, Twisted and Wide
both sides

Pigeon
Thigh Stretch

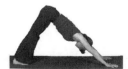 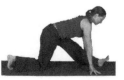 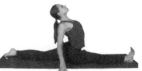 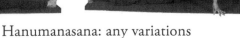 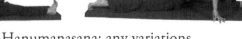

Down Dog
enjoy your breath

Ardha Hanumanasana
(Runner's Lunge)

Hanumanasana: any variations

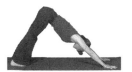

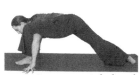

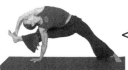

< VINYASA >

Down Dog
enjoy your breath

Lunge with leg behind shoulder
Optional: Vishvamitrasana

Uttanasana
enjoy your breath

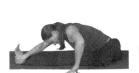

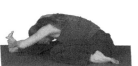

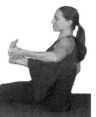

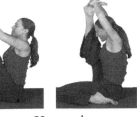

Janu Sirsasana

Triang Mukhaikapada
Paschimottanasana

Krounchasana prep or Krounchasana

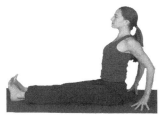

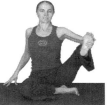

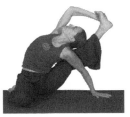

Dandasana
(Staff Pose)

Surya Yantrasana (Sundial Pose)

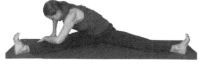

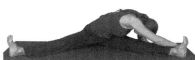

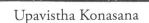

Parsva Upavistha Konasana

Upavistha Konasana

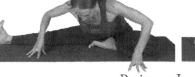

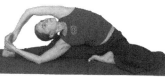

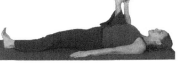
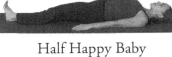

Parivrtta Janu Sirsasana
repeat to go deeper

Half Happy Baby

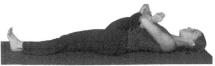

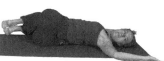

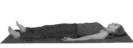

Supine Pigeon
or Thread the Needle

Finishing Twist

Hug and Rock

Savasana

Purity and Flow

The Virtues: Purity, Clarity, Focus, Flow.

Coming together with Shakti, flowing with sensitivity.
Cleanse and release, refocus, and align with the Divine current of Grace.

The Focus: Twists

The Apex: Dhanurasana, Kali Thigh Stretch, Parivrtta Trikonasana, Bound Parivrtta Parsvakonasana, Bound Parsvakonasana and Trikonasana

SEQUENCE:

Surya Namaskar with Lunge Twist

Surya Namaskar with Anjaneyasana

Uttanasana Shoulder Opener

Vinyasa

Crescent to Vira III

Parsvakonasana > Trikonasana > Ardha Chandrasana > Parivrtta Ardha Chandrasana

Garudasana

Vinyasa

Parivrtta Utkatasana

Parivrtta Parsvakonasana (x2 – bound variation optional)

Kali Thigh Stretch

Dhanurasana (x2)

Parsvottanasana

Parivrtta Hasta Padangusthasana

Vinyasa

Parsvakonasana and Trikonasana (bound variations optional)

Anjaneyasana thigh stretch

Twisted pigeon

Parsvottanasana > Parivrtta Trikonasana

Uttanasana

144

Parivrtta Malasana

Uttanasana

Janu Sirsasana

Ardha Matsyendrasana

Parivrtta Upavistha Konasana

Baddha Konasana

Parivrtta Supta Padangusthasana

Savasana

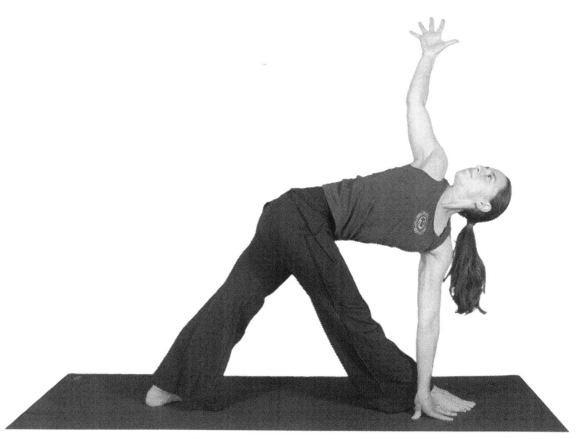

Parivrtta Trikonasana (Revolved Triangle Pose)

Purity and Flow

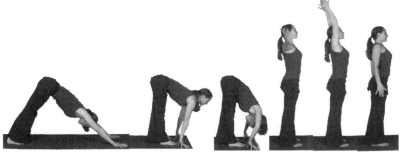

< SURYA NAMASKAR - SUN SALUTATION >

< VINYASA >

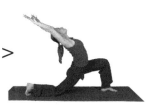

Anjaneyasana

< VINYASA >

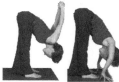

Uttanasana
shoulder stretch

< VINYASA >

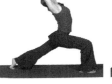

Crescent Lunge > Vira III
both sides

< VINYASA >

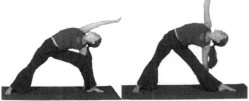

FLOW: Parsvakonasana > Trikonasana > Ardha Chandrasana
repeat FLOW on other side

< VINYASA >

< VINYASA >

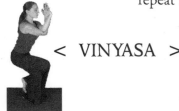

Garudasana
(Eagle Pose)

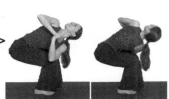

Parivrtta Utkatasana

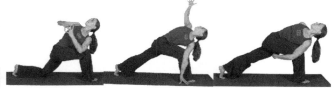

Parivrtta Parsvakonasana: any variations
repeat twice on each side to go deeper (optional bind)

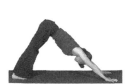
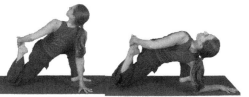
< VINYASA >
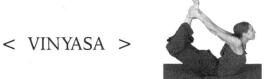

Down Dog
enjoy your breath

Kali Thigh Stretch

Dhanurasana
(Bow Pose)

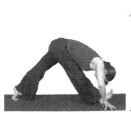
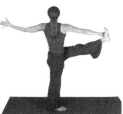
< VINYASA >
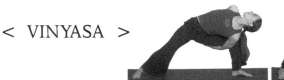

Parsvattonasana
variation

Parivrtta Hasta
Padangusthasana

Parsvakonasana > Trikonasana
Optional: bound variations
both sides

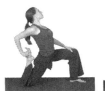
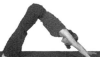
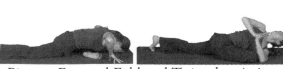
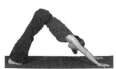

Anjaneyasana
Thigh Stretch

Breathe.

Pigeon: Forward Fold and Twisted variation
both sides

Breathe.

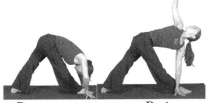

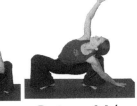
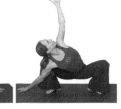

Parsvottanasana > Parivrtta
Trikonasana both sides

Parivrtta Malasana
(Revolved Garland Pose)

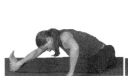

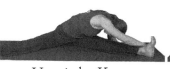
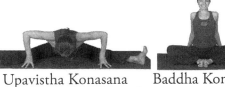

Janu Sirsasana

Ardha
Matsyendrasana

Parsva Upavistha Konasana

Upavistha Konasana

Baddha Konasana

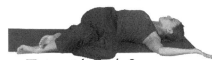
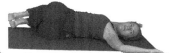

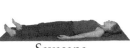

Twist with Eagle Legs

Finishing Twist

Hug and Rock

Savasana

Waves of Pulsation

The Virtues: Harmonious pulsation through Gratitude and Generosity, Receptivity and Reciprocity.

The Focus: Forward Bends (and optional Inversions)

The Apex: Hanumanasana, Sirsasana, Sarvangasana

SEQUENCE:

Uttanasana

Dragon Lunge with twist

Uttanasana

Vinyasa

Parsvottanasana

Vinyasa

Anjaneyasana

Runner's Lunge

Vira II to Trikonasana

Pigeon

Parsvakonasana to Ardha Chandrasana (optional Ardha Chandra Chapasana)

Standing splits

Vinyasa

Pigeon Thigh Stretch

Uttanasana

Setu Bandha / Urdhva Dhanurasana (optional)

Uttanasana

Vinyasa

Hanumanasana (x3 variations)

Pigeon forward and twisted

Uttanasana

Janu Sirsasana

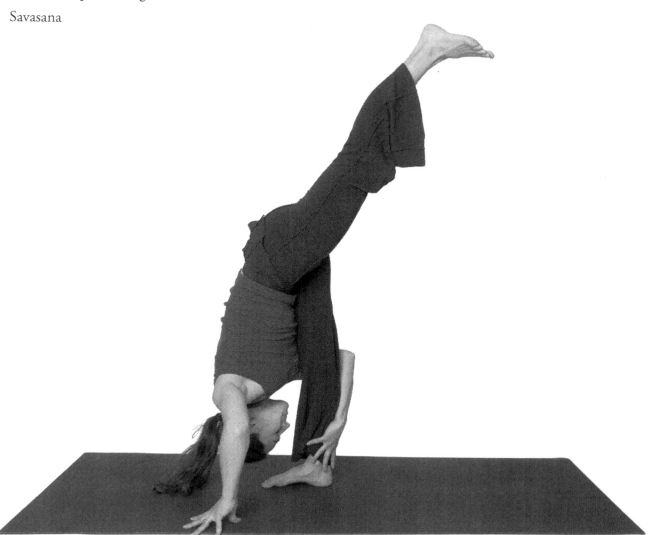

Urdhva Prasarita Ekapadasana (Standing Split Pose)

Waves of Pulsation

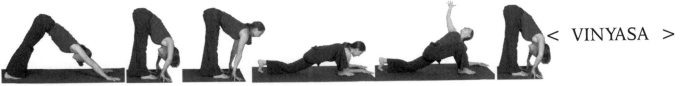 **< VINYASA >**

Down Dog
move as you like

Uttanasana
pulse with your breath

Dragon Lunge Twist
both sides

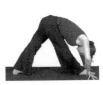 **< VINYASA >** 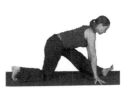 **< VINYASA >**

Parsvottanasana
both sides

Anjaneyasana
both sides

Ardha Hanumanasana
(Runner's Lunge)

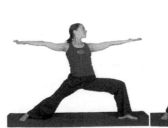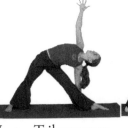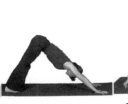 **< VINYASA >**

FLOW: Virabhadrasana II > Trikonasana
repeat FLOW on other side

Pigeon Forward Fold

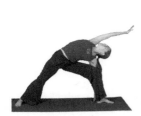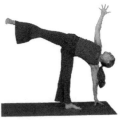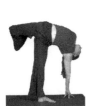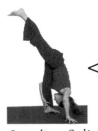 **< VINYASA >**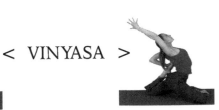

FLOW: Parsvakonasana > Ardha Chandra > Chapasana
repeat FLOW on other side

Standing Splits
both sides

Pigeon
Thigh Stretch

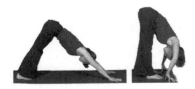 Pause in Tadasana
or Child's Pose

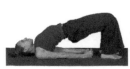

Breathe. Feel. Be.

Setu Bandha
Sarvangasana

Optional:
Urdhva Dhanurasana

< VINYASA >

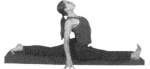

Hanumanasana: any variations

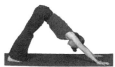

Breathe.

Pigeon Forward Fold and Twisted
both sides

Janu Sirsasana

Agnistambhasana
(Fire-Log Pose)

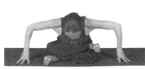

Agnistambhasana
Forward Fold

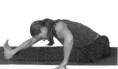

Janu Sirsasana
again ~ go deeper.

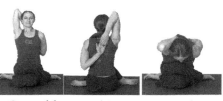

Gomukhasana (Cow Face Pose)
Optional: Forward Fold

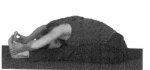

Pachimottanasana
(Seated Forward Bend)

PLEASE DO HEADSTAND AND SHOULDERSTAND ONLY IF THEY ARE ALREADY A REGULAR PART OF YOUR PRACTICE.

These are best learned in class, not from a book.
Use of blankets in Sarvangasana is encouraged.

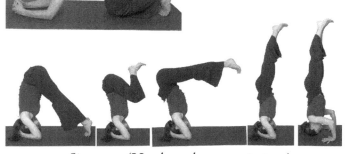

Sirsasana (Headstand: any variations)

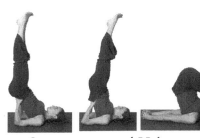

Sarvangasana and Halasana
(Shoulderstand and Plow)

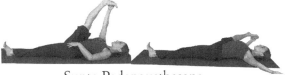

Supta Padangusthasana

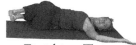

Finishing Twist

Hug and Rock

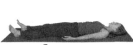

Savasana

Cradle of Healing (Restorative)

The Virtues: Nurturing, Acceptance, and Healing.

The Focus: Restorative Yoga and Gentle Stretches

The Apex: Viparita Kanari (Legs Up the Wall) or Supported Shoulderstand

Note: With the restorative poses, start with a 2 minute hold and work up to 5 or more minutes. Be sure that you are comfortable, take your time in transitions, and subtly apply alignment even as you release and relax.

SEQUENCE:

Supta Baddha Konasana

Supported Child's Pose

Adho Mukha Svanasana (Down Dog)

Uttanasana

Parsvottanasana

Anjaneyasana

Parighasana

Uttanasana

Supported Chest Opener

Supported Child's Pose

Adho Mukha Svanasana

Pigeon (or Thread the Needle)

Setu Bandha (Bridge)

Windshield Wipers

Hamstring Hug

Supported Twist

Supported Child

Viparita Kanari

or Supported Shoulderstand

Savasana

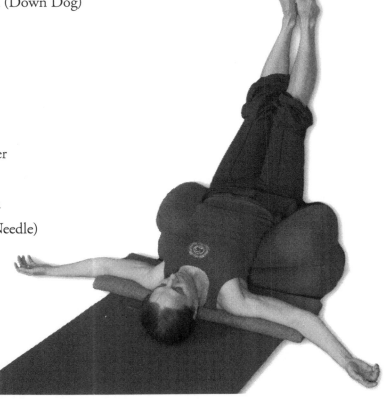

Supported Shoulderstand (against wall)

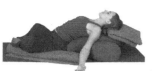
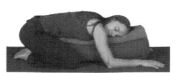
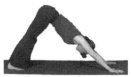

Supta Baddha Konasana
(Reclining Bound Angle Pose)

Supported Child's Pose

Down Dog
move as you like

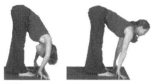
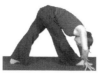
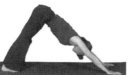
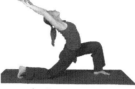

Uttanasana
pulse with your breath

Parsvottanasana
both sides

Anjaneyasana
both sides

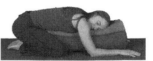

Parighasana (Gate Keeper Pose)
go to both sides on each side

Supported Chest
Opener

Supported Child's Pose

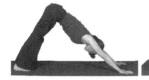
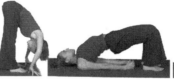

Windshield Wipers
slow, with your breath

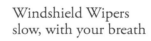

Pigeon Forward Fold
both sides

Setu Bandha
Sarvangasana

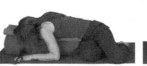

Supported Twist both sides

Supported Child's Pose

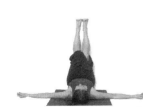
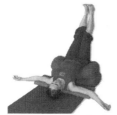
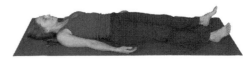

Breathe. Feel. Be.

Viparita Kanari (Legs Up the Wall Pose) or Supported Shoulderstand

Other Practices

EAGLE EYES

Attending to the health of your eyes is an essential part of practicing. We tend to use our eyes in the same ways repeatedly, such as staring at a computer screen or reading a book. So to keep them healthy with optimal circulation, you want to spend a few minutes each day to use all the muscles in the eyes as well as allow them to rest. The following exercise is one way to do this.

Take a deep breath to center yourself.

Sit or stand, grounded and steady.

Rub your palms together to warm your hands and activate the chakras—energy centers—in your palms. (You bring energy there with your focus, and this energy interacts in a healing way with your eyes while you do the exercise).

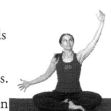

Take your hands wide to either side of you, palms facing each other, hands even with the height of your eyes and just on the edge of your periphery.

Look from side to side with your eyes, back and forth between your palms.

Take your hands back toward the center, see if you can feel energy between them, and then out diagonally, one up one down, and look back and forth between the two.

Take your hands back towards center and then to the opposite diagonal.

Gaze back and forth.

Remember to breathe.

Then take your hands so the palms almost touch, about 4 to 6 inches in front of your nose, and shift your gaze from your fingertips to a focal point in the distance. You can play with different distances, going back and forth between focal points and the tips of your fingers.

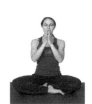

Take a deep breath as you rub your hands together again.

Then, place your palms over your eyes and close them.

With your hands cupping over your eyes, the palm chakras sending healing energy into them, take your eyes in a big infinity shape, tracing a sideways figure 8 beneath your eyelids. Up, around, down, center, up the other side, around, down, center, and so on. Go around at least a few times, then go the other direction.

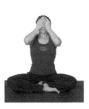

When you're done, let your eyes rest back in the darkness for a couple of deep breaths.

154

Pranayama and Meditation

Meditation and breath practices (pranayama) are integral elements of practicing yoga and can be woven into an asana practice.

These are covered in the next stage of your Training.

Other Forms of Exercise

As a Dragon Rider, you want to be able to run, jump, swim, climb trees, fly and do pretty much anything else you need or want with your body as you adventure in life and help save the world.

You can apply what you learn in yoga to any activity.

Stay strong. Work out. Play. Expand the boundaries of your capacity.

All of this is part of being a Dragon Rider and moving towards Mastery: exploring different experiences and cultivating skill in every element of life.

The Power of Play

Play. Really, yoga is profound, Divine play. Lila. Joy connects us to the Divine.

Be creative in your expression of it. Empower your practice with play.

There are so many ways! Here are a few ideas that you might run with, sparking new ideas of your own.

Dancing: When you get your groove on, it puts you in the natural flow of Shakti. You breathe, you move, you're one with the music. This is an excellent practice in flow and pulsation.

Swings: Swinging on swings at a playground can be fun, somewhat simulating the feeling of riding a Dragon. Think *Whooomp. Whooomp. Whooomp.* As the wings of your Dragon keep time with the swing. It can also be a good little workout if you play with balance, alignment, and what it's like to be at the bottom of a pendulum.

Singing: Let your song be heard! Play in the realm of sound and make beauty there. More on that in the Initiation of Resonance . . .

Drawing/Creating Art: Explore the limitless expressions of art and find lila (Divine play) in the making, enjoying, and discovering.

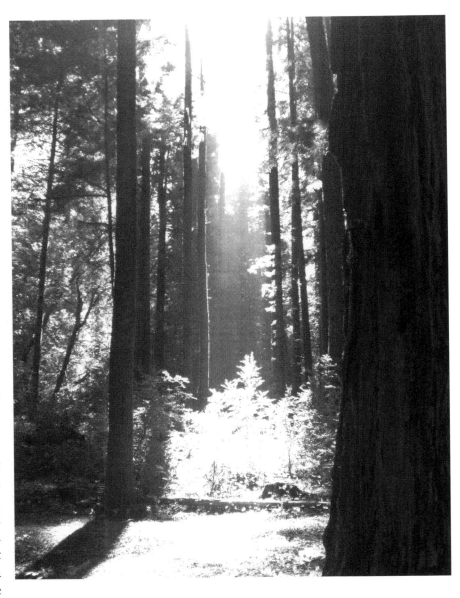

Trees: Spending time with trees is grounding, healing, and a wonderful way to develop sensitivity and connection to Nature. If you are sensitive and listen, the trees will tell you things. You can get messages or specific feelings with different trees. Hug them, climb them, sit beneath them, or simply admire them.

Hiking: Go on an excursion. Pack provisions, take a friend or go solo. Know the land you walk. Sing mantra as you go. Observe in detail and see what feelings come— realize that Nature is a part of yourself. Run the hills or flats to get more exercise. Stand on rocks, sing to rivers, swim in lakes. Smell the flowers and laugh with the sun. Invent new ways to do yoga in relationship with the natural world you discover.

Be freely who you are, in harmonious relationship with all around you,
in whatever way you are inspired.

This is living yoga—awareness and union in each moment, in motion and in stillness.

Closing and Honoring

Integration, transition, and contemplation

Like any ritual, like any practice that creates mindful patterns, there is an intentional closing.

The end of each asana practice session is your time to integrate, transition, and contemplate any insights that come up for you.

This brings a balancing energy, and helps you to carry the benefits of your practice with you so you can live your yoga off the mat. Transitioning in this way, from mindful practice to mindful living, is an integral part of being a Dragon Rider—it brings a vigilant awareness to every moment.

Taking a moment to honor your path—your dedication to your highest self—is a key action in linking the transformative power of your yoga practice with the rest of your life.

Savasana

Savasana (pronounced "shavasana," remember) literally translates as "corpse pose" and signifies the end of the practice and a time of transition, as well as a fresh start when you come out of it.

It is one of the most difficult yoga poses to do fully.

Why?

Well, because totally relaxing and yet staying fully present is not something most of us know how to do. Yet this pose is one of the most beneficial, so it's worth giving the practice of mindful relaxation your best . . . er . . . effort.

Some people fall asleep in Savasana. This is because their body says, "Oh, we're lying down and relaxing, eh? Guess it's time for a nap." Which makes sense when you consider that sleeping may be the only time many people actually relax.

Others have a very difficult time letting go, and really have to work to release tension in their bodies and minds.

But for the majority of people, the hardest part is staying mindfully focused while all this relaxation is happening. The mind wanders easily. It's a simple fact.

SAVASANA ITSELF IS A YOGA PRACTICE.

It's a good thing yoga is a practice, not something you're expected to do perfectly right off the bat—or ten years into it for that matter. In fact, you're perfect just as you are, so don't worry about it. Just keep doing your very best every time and you will continue to improve.

One thing you should keep in mind about Savasana is that it isn't a collapse. There's a difference between relaxing and collapsing. Relaxing is mindful; there is an inner fullness which the outer body, muscles, bones, organs, and so on, are held by as they soften. Collapse is not supported, and does not allow the circulation of blood, lymph, Prana, and breath that is so necessary for optimal healing.

When you do Savasana, start by aligning your body as best you can. Then feel the brightness within—feel how full of life you are! Allow that inner fullness to keep you buoyant from within, then drape your outer body over it. While your inner body remains spacious, let your skin drape, your bones be heavy, your organs rest. Settle into your back body.

And then, in this relaxed yet illuminated state, breathe.

Feel your breath enter and leave. Notice how your body pulses with the breath and how that feels. Notice that by focusing on certain areas of your body with your breath, these parts of your body relax further.

Any time your mind wanders, gently and lovingly bring it back to the breath. The practice of Savasana brings you the most benefits when you are present in the moment.

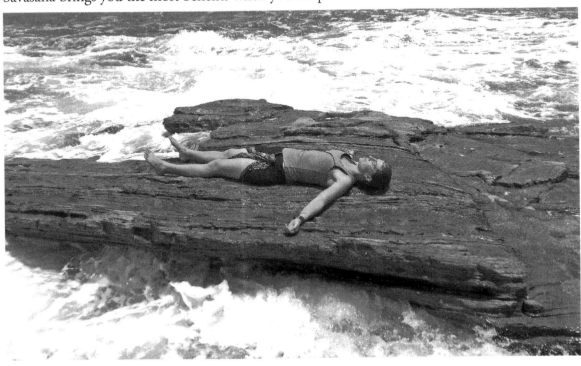

What are the benefits of Savasana?

There are many. Here are just a few:

- ~ It is one of the best possible ways to de-stress and reduce anxiety.
- ~ It distributes blood and other vital fluids and nutrients evenly throughout the body.
- ~ It allows the body time to recover and assimilate the myriad benefits of your yoga practice.
- ~ It calms the brain and body, and it helps to lower blood pressure.
- ~ It can help reduce headaches, insomnia and fatigue.

There's more, but aren't those reasons enough?

Do Savasana at the end of every yoga practice. Though seated meditation is sometimes an appropriate alternative, in my experience Savasana is what the body, mind, and spirit crave after a yoga practice. It is very important to be still and mindful, and to relax and breathe as a transition between your asana practice and the rest of your day. Don't skip it.

Savasana can also be done on its own, though even one or two sun salutations or a short practice can help to get your circulation flowing, increasing the benefits of your relaxation.

Closing Meditation and Blessing

At the end of your practice, allow time to be still and reflect. Feel your breath. Ground yourself. Notice the shift your practice has created in you. This might be a few moments, it might be many minutes or even a long meditation.

Give yourself time to close your practice, even if it is just one mindful breath. This helps to settle your energy and focus so you can continue to benefit from your practice as you leave your mat and go about your life.

Finish with a blessing and an OM. You may also want to bow your head in honor.

Namaste

Namaste is the traditional word uttered at the end of a yoga practice. It is said from teacher to student and from student to teacher. You can say it to yourself and to the world around you. *Namaste* is also used as a greeting in India, and is found in various forms in other cultures. It has many uses and implications, but the basic meaning is, "The Spirit in me bows to the Spirit in you."

Here is one of my favorite descriptions of *Namaste*:

> *I honor the place in you in which the entire Universe dwells.*
> *I honor the place in you which is of love, of truth, of light, and of peace.*
> *When you are in that place in you, and I am in that place in me, we are one.*

—Author Unknown

Integrating the Fourth Initiation

Practice.

Practice nearly every day, even for just five or ten minutes.

Practice so you know your body, and so that it feels good to be embodied.

Practice. Learn from what it has to teach you.

Practice in the way that is best for your body in each changing moment.

Practice with devotion to awakening and delight.

Practice.

Get on your mat and Ride your Dragon.

The Fifth Initiation:
Clarity

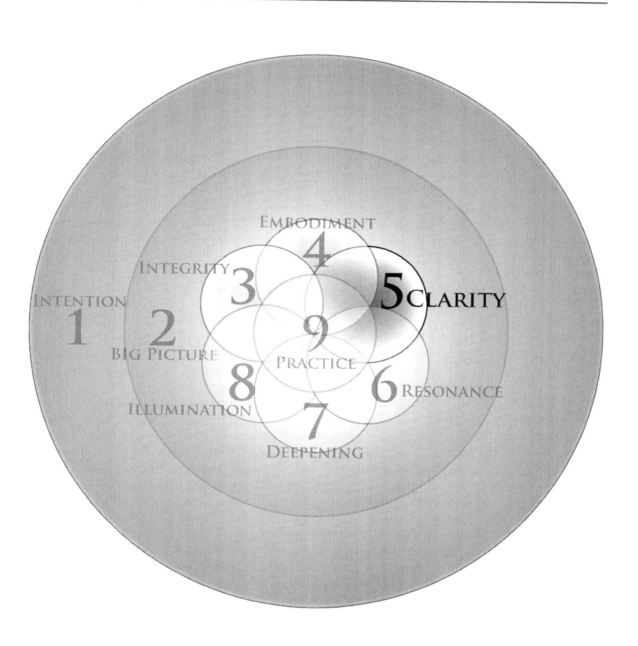

Cultivate Focus and Contentment

Think for a moment about some of the most famous super-human sci-fi or fantasy movie characters: the Jedis from *Star Wars,* Neo in *The Matrix,* even Aragorn from *The Lord of the Rings.*

What drove these characters to triumph over the seemingly impossible?

Focus, will, and an ability to find a degree of inner peace through self-mastery—even when they were experiencing very human feelings such as fear, anger, love, and the need to survive.

They also all had a very clear purpose. Laser-clear intent. That is what helped them focus.

It helped that they were highly motivated too. The fate of the world resting on their shoulders would do that.

What about you?

If you knew that the fate of the world was in your hands, would you do what it takes to Master yourself?

Would you summon the will to focus and do the work to clear clutter from your mind and emotions? Would you be willing to soften your pride and devote yourself to becoming a more loving, pure, peaceful person than you have ever been in any of your lifetimes?

Do you realize that the fate of the world *does* rest in your hands? At least in part . . .

WHY IT MATTERS

One of the most important abilities for happiness, harmony, and success as a human being is to be able to focus and reach a place of deep contentment.

Clearing your mind and choosing your thoughts (rather than letting them bombard you) is a primary theme in yoga. The practices we'll explore in this section, namely meditation and pranayama, are designed to calm your mind and harmonize your feelings.

Focus and inner peace are essential for Dragon Riders.

Why?

Well, first consider this: If you are so powerful that what you think manifests immediately, you want to be sure you can focus on what you *want* to happen, rather than be randomly creating fearful thoughts or chaos.

Although, that whole instant-manifestation thing really doesn't show up on a regular basis unless you are able to precisely focus your intent.

Still . . . even if it isn't instant, thoughts become things, so it's good to be able to choose thoughts that create a world of harmony and beauty, don't you think?

Second, let's look at the necessity of finding contentment.

Yes, it feels good, cultivates balance and good will, basically bringing you into a place where you are able to flow gracefully with whatever life brings.

However, the alternative, especially for Dragon Riders or others who gain great power, is very dangerous.

Think about it: If you wield power without the balance of love and wisdom (both of which are present in profound peace) then you've got problems.

Pretty much all of the imbalance, war, and tragedy created by the human race has come due to the actions of people with power who were lacking the key factors of love and contentment.

They acted instead out of fear and the desire to dominate, which doesn't make a person feel warm and fuzzy inside. Sure, they have focus, but it is false and misplaced. Without a foundation of goodness, clarity becomes confused, and inner conflict eats away at the emotions and physical body.

Which really isn't a great way to live or influence the world.

Contentment can only come when you are aligned with your purpose, with integrity, with clear intent to live a life that is informed by the highest elements of love, wisdom, and power in complete balance.

Which might sound difficult.

However, that deep abiding peace that your heart seeks can be found more easily than you may think.

The secret is remembering that it has been there all the time, has never left you, and never will.

Here are some ways to do so.

Meditation

Meditation's proven benefits have been hailed by scientists, the deeply spiritual, successful business people, and busy parents alike. It has been scientifically established as a more effective approach to pain reduction than morphine. It brings peace of mind and contentment.

There are individuals from all walks of life who use this ancient practice to find equanimity in modern times, and it is one of the most important aspects of life for millions of people.

Why is meditation such a big deal? Well, it is a conscious connection with the Source of who you are. A connection that helps you remember the big picture and let go of worries. It is a choice to be in the here and now, the magic moment where the pressures of past and future dissolve into the simplicity of be-ing.

This Initiation is simply a starting point, with a few ways to begin or enhance your meditation practice. More will be given in the Initiations of Resonance and Illumination.

The Benefits of Meditation Include:

- ⁓ Decrease in stress and all its side effects
- ⁓ Increase in focus and calm
- ⁓ Increase in mental and emotional capacity
- ⁓ Higher quality of circulation and breathing
- ⁓ Healing on every level
- ⁓ Brings peace of mind, calm contentedness, and happiness
- ⁓ Helps you understand yourself and the world
- ⁓ Expands your capacity to receive and give love
- ⁓ Gives a profound sense of oneness

THE MANY FORMS OF MEDITATION

Practicing meditation is perhaps the most effective way to find peace and balance in your life. There are many forms and approaches to meditation, but the basic idea is to calm and clear the mind while entering fully into the moment. When your mind and body are steady, the light of your heart is more fully revealed and a feeling of deep peace is experienced.

Traditionally, meditation is done sitting still, with exquisite posture, so that the spine has its natural curves and energy and breath can move freely. In general, many of the most profound meditative experiences happen in seated meditation.

However, you can bring a meditative quality to movement, such as in yoga practice, or any activity where you immerse your focus completely. Dancing, working, chopping carrots, watching the clouds, petting a cat, or any other seemingly ordinary experience can be a meditation if your awareness is totally absorbed in the present.

Walking meditation can be wonderful as well. Every step is mindful.

Though all forms of moving meditation are valuable, stilling the body is a great way to help still the mind. And, let's be realistic, when it comes to calming the relentlessness of thoughts, we need all the help we can get.

Don't be frustrated when your mind keeps turning.
This does not mean you are failing at meditation.
It means you're a human being.

THE CIRCUS OF THE MIND

If you sometimes get discouraged when you meditate because you find that your mind simply will not be still, don't be hard on yourself. This is normal. The mind is designed to think. It's good at it, and you have spent your entire life encouraging it to do just that. It is natural that it will take some practice to get the thoughts to take even a brief rest.

The game is to find the gaps between your thoughts. You gather your awareness and focus it on one thing, such as the breath, or a mantra, or a feeling.

As thoughts come through, you just let them go again, without holding onto them or following them. I find it helpful to be gently amused by my chattering mind while I meditate, and to keep returning to my focus over and over with loving patience. There are many different things you can focus on in meditation: the point is that you actually *have* a focus, rather than allowing the mind to run amok.

Though your mind will do all kinds of tricks for you while you encourage it to be quiet, if you are consistent with your practice and as you continue to refocus as many times as necessary to be in the moment, meditating will get easier. It is part of the process.

FUELING THE ECSTATIC FIRE

It is important to fuel your meditation practice with intention. To maintain your practice, know why you are doing it.

If you meditate because you think you should, chances are it will lack enjoyment and won't be much of a priority. Anything that is forced loses its potency and can quickly become a chore.

Meditation is meant to be an energizing, enlivening, sweet connection of deep love and peace. Don't let it get dry by forgetting what it's all about.

Remember, as a Dragon Rider you are on the path to Mastery of the self. Let this help you bring a deep meaning to your meditation practice.

When you choose to meditate from a deep desire to awaken from the feeling of being separate from the Divine, or because you want to find freedom and peace, then you will make time for it. It will become so important that you will carve space in even the busiest of days to get your hit of this purest of highs. With this kind of motivation, meditation will become something you crave, something you want to do, and your practice will be very rewarding.

THE START OF SOMETHING GREAT

If you don't already have a meditation practice, or if you have fallen out of practice, you might be asking, *So, how do I start?* Or, you might be thinking, *I want to meditate, but I don't have time.* The response to both of those thoughts is the same.

You make time for yourself.

Decide that it is important enough to get up 20 minutes earlier, or take 10 minutes of your lunch break, or 15 minutes before bed. Whenever it is best for you, set aside what time you can. It is nice if you practice meditation at the same time each day, but if this isn't realistic, it's okay. Just make sure you meditate at some point.

It may be a good idea to start with shorter periods of time. Try sitting still for 5 or 10 minutes. Then go to 15. You will find yourself naturally wanting to sit for longer periods of time, but it's nice to start off easy so you don't feel discouraged or obligated.

When thoughts come through, just let them go again. Think of your mind as an exuberant puppy or a small child who is easily distracted. With love and infinite patience for yourself, keep returning your awareness to your focus—whatever your focus happens to be for that meditation (the breath, a mantra, a visualization, etc.)

Once your meditation practice takes shape, you will feel the benefits and it will naturally become the most important thing for you to do. Even if you only have 5 minutes, find stillness and some measure of inner calm, and you will notice the difference in your life.

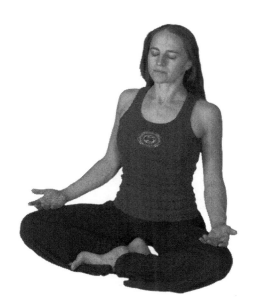

The Beauty of Breath Meditation

Focusing on your breath is one of the simplest and sweetest ways to meditate. Feel how your breath moves. Receive the breath as a gift.

Don't get caught up in the tangle of your thoughts. Instead, as a wise man once told me, "Think, *Just this breath.*"

The Beauty of Breath

Sit beautifully. Settle into your pelvis.
Grow taller in your spine.
Allow a spaciousness to expand within you.
Notice how your breath fills that space.

For the next few minutes,
Simply breathe.
Be a witness to the beauty of your breath,
It is the movement of life within.
Feel it as a gift from the Source of who you are.
Let it be a wonder.

When thoughts come, just let them go again,
And keep bringing your awareness back to
The beauty of your breath.

Close your eyes and enjoy the peace
That your breath brings.

Happy Meditation

My beloved, Casey, likes to practice what he calls "happy meditation." He thinks of a memory or thought that brings joy, then stays with the feeling of happiness, letting the thought float away. I love seeing him sit with his eyes closed and a peaceful smile on his face.

You can do this with any feeling: love, gratitude, peace, compassion, forgiveness.

Any attribute that brings light and healing to you is worthy of your attention.

Happy Meditation

Align your spine and sit beautifully.
Take a few breaths to feel your body.
Feel your breath.

Then, think of a moment in your life that brought you great happiness
Let the feeling of joy fill you.
If it begins to fade, think of another happy memory.
Let the memories bring the feeling to you so strongly
That you can simply stay with the feeling of joy,
And let the image of the memory dissolve.

Close your eyes and breathe here,
In the warmth of your heart,
In the fullness of this feeling.

Walking Meditation

The idea of walking meditation, just like other meditations, is to be fully present. You can bring such awareness to the way you walk, your surroundings, and the moment itself, that this practice can create a heightened state of connection and peace.

My first experience with walking meditation was at a yoga teacher-training in Baja, Mexico. Each morning we got up super early, did a short asana practice, and then went out to the beach for walking meditation.

I would place my feet slowly, mindfully, listening to the waves crash on the shore. I would feel the subtleties of each step, and often would close my eyes or even walk backwards to shift my perspective.

LEARNING WALKING MEDITATION

The way I learned walking meditation was basically to learn how to walk again—very slowly. Now, it doesn't have to be the same for you, and you don't have to do walking meditation super-slow motion, but it's helpful to start that way and train yourself to stay focused; then you can speed it up.

One way to do this is to stand with your knees bent, then pick up one foot, play with the balance, and place it down very slowly. Walk in place like this in slow motion, then start moving forward (or backward, or sideways) in full mindfulness.

Another way to learn walking meditation is simply to walk and notice as much as you can in the moment.

- Can you feel every part of your body and the way your feet move?
- What does your breath feel like?
- Can you create more space inside and let your breath move deeper?
- What sounds do you hear?
- What colors do you see?
- What does the air feel like on your skin?

WAYS TO FOCUS WHILE PRACTICING WALKING MEDITATION

There are some truly beautiful ways to gather and hone your focus while doing this practice. Here are some ideas for you:

- Notice as much as you can in each moment (see questions above for cues).
- Think about planting lotus flowers with your feet as you take each step.
- Use a mantra, such as *Om Namah Shivaya*, or *Om Shanti*. (We'll go over these mantras and many others in the Initiation on Resonance).
- Work with an intention or affirmation, repeating it like a mantra.
- Feel each breath fully.
- Think of all that you're grateful for—see how long you can keep this up!

Though getting outside in the fresh air is ideal, you can do this on a treadmill as well. Or you can pace up and down your hallway, or anywhere else for that matter, if going outside isn't an option.

Also, if you have gentle-natured or obedient four legged friends along for your walk, you can still do this. Just stay calm and in the moment whenever you need to help them remember what they need to do. Don't let yourself get pulled out of your center by your companions (literally or energetically). Instead, have full patience with them and yourself.

Pranayama

Every Dragon would agree that breath is life, and it connects us to all that lives around us.

This is why one of the main focuses of yoga is the breath, including the practice of pranayama.

Pranayama is often referred to as "breath control," however I much prefer to consider it a "co-created dance" with your breath.

To me, the concept of control calls in the hardened attitude of domination and separation with one being in control over another.

But we're speaking of Nature in one of her most essential forms—the movement of life! For pranayama to bring joy and contentment, doesn't it make sense to deeply honor the relationship between yourself and your breath? And, when you think about it . . . where does the breath end and you begin?

In pranayama you are directing your breath to dance in specific ways and to move as you ask, yet because the breath contains the essence of life, this dance is one of great respect and care.

So much of yoga is about the breath, for breath is infused with Prana (also known as Chi or Qi), which is literally the energy of life—Shakti dancing within.

Prana pulsates within every part of you—down to every single cell—and all of life.

When you honor your breath and your intention is to invite Prana to create a state of harmony within you, the rewards of health and happiness are bountiful!

The physical benefits are many, clearing toxins and bringing increased circulation and nutrients to all systems and parts of the body. As you clear toxins and enhance vitality physically, pranayama also moves toxic or stagnant thoughts and emotions. And by dissipating these thoughts and emotions, you end up with a spacious mind and peaceful state of being.

Pranayama, along with many other practices of yoga, is credited with bestowing long life and enhanced states of meditation.

Can you recall the feeling of your breath really opening up in a yoga pose? Or the shifting of your mind and emotions into a state of peace when you pause and just turn your focus to your breath?

Whether you are dancing with the breath in a seated practice of pranayama, or flowing with your breath in an active asana practice on your mat, this attitude of co-participation allows you to stay humble and in remembrance that Prana weaves a bigger energy into your life.

Your intention is so important when you do yoga—including and especially with pranayama—because this dance of breath manifests the feelings of your intention. For instance, if you are holding an attitude that is hardened, forced, angry, or fearful when you do yoga or practice pranayama, the Prana gets agitated and it can worsen the difficulties you're dealing with, even to the point of being harmful.

Just as a misaligned yoga pose can increase risk of injury, a misaligned attitude or technique in pranayama can do harm to the body, mind and/or emotions. Don't mess around with your breath—if you feel irritation or there is any kind of pain, release the technique gently but immediately and return to allowing your breath to move naturally.

Some people have trauma associated with the breath and have to go very slowly as they learn pranayama, but most people can steadily incorporate the practices more and more into their lives.

That said, so long as you use pranayama respectfully and mindfully, it is generally very healing, rejuvenating, and soothing. It is also an important aspect to enrich and develop your yoga and meditation practices.

Keep in mind that no matter what feelings you are experiencing when you start your practice, if you have the attitude that you are turning towards the light of illumination, intending to transform those feelings by opening to a bigger energy as you practice, then your breath will take you there.

Breath is the bridge between intention and manifestation. Breath carries great power, moving energy in the cycle of creation. It is the constant interweaving of Individual and Universal, and therefore brings the Universal influence and Individual intent together to form reality.

Practicing Pranayama

There are many types of pranayama, and it is best to dive into this practice while being led in person by a teacher. But if you're practicing on your own, here are several general things to keep in mind.

1. Always begin by simply observing your natural breath without any objective other than to focus on how you feel as the Prana moves through your inhale and exhale. By first honoring the natural pulsation of your breath as it is, and opening to receive the breath as a gift of Grace, you will be more in harmony when you begin different techniques in the form of pranayama.

2. Just as in yoga, you never want to force or strain. If you feel your body tighten or resist when you're doing pranayama, soften and allow your breath to lead, rather than your mind.

   If this softening doesn't melt the tension, release the technique you were working with and simply return to watching the natural breath with the intention of being sensitive and sweet.

3. Your posture has influence over how your breath moves and how freely the Prana can flow within you. If you are aligned in a beautiful seated position, optimal circulation

carries the Prana through your body and your experience is enhanced.

If you are slumped, misaligned, or in pain, it obviously restricts the experience. This is why asana practice is such an integral part of yoga, because it helps you learn to align in ways that feel good and offer Grace in the dance of pranayama, meditation, and every other part of life.

Also, though there are some techniques that instruct breathing through the mouth, all of the techniques included here are meant to be done through the nostrils. If you find restriction or blockage in the nostrils (one or both sides), don't force. Ujjayi breath can help to clear excess mucus, as can using a neti pot to irrigate your nasal passages with a warm saline solution. If you're really struggling, simply use the Slow, Deep Breathing technique. (Ujjayi and the Slow, Deep Breathing techniques are both outlined in this section.)

Pranayama can be done before meditation, at the beginning of a yoga practice, at the end before Savasana, or during an asana practice that is more inwardly directed, such as a hip opening or forward bending sequence. Or, pranayama can simply be practiced on its own.

About the Bandhas

Bandhas are translated as blocks or bindings. In the context of pranayama they are referred to as "locks." These are used to create a container for Prana within the main portion of the body, between the root chakra and throat chakra.

These bandhas are very subtle, and therefore can be elusive. Some schools of yoga use these locks in extreme ways. I prefer to use them in more refined ways, which I find to be just as effective.

The main three bandhas that are used to respectfully hold and build energy within the body are as follows:

> *Mula Bandha*
> *Uddiyana Bandha*
> *Jalandhara Bandha*

Conveniently, when you apply some refined alignment of yoga, you end up creating these bandhas.

Mula Bandha tones the pelvic floor, and Uddiyana Bandha tones the lower belly. Combined they create a bottom for the container of energy. This happens when you first widen your inner thighs back and apart, and then (keeping the thighs rooted back) strongly scoop your tail bone forward. Try it and see if you feel the uplifted feeling in your lower belly and pelvic floor.

These two lower bandhas create an upward flow of energy. Mula Bandha as been described as a very subtle lifting, like slowly sucking on a straw. You can purse your lips and very softly inhale to get a sense of this feeling.

Jalandhara Bandha is the roof of the container, creating an energetic boundary above the throat chakra that lets the energy build within. This can be envisioned as a solid boundary that contains all energy, or a thin one that allows some energy to rise.

A subtle binding can be created using intention and aligning thus: Use your inhale to lift your heart and take your shoulders back, then—starting with your head slightly lifted—move your chin gently downward to tone the throat and bring your head slightly back from your jaw. You should feel a firmness in your throat, but you can still breathe easily and there is no strain.

When do you use these bandhas? Well, Mula Bandha and Uddiyana Bandha are naturally found in many yoga poses, as well as many pranayama exercises. Jalandhara Bandha is used in some pranayama practices as well.

But not all.

For instance, in pranayama you would generally use all three bandhas for Ujjayi and Nadi Shodhana, but not for Kapalabhati (all of which are included in this section).

In asana, you would use the lower two bandhas for most poses (but women would be good to avoid them during menstruation because they draw energy up in the pelvis). Jalandhara bandha naturally occurs in poses like Shoulderstand.

If you're still finding the bandhas elusive to understand, no worries. You're not alone. This is something that can be learned over time, and is not essential to apply to get the rewards of pranayama.

Preparing for Pranayama

Remember, before you start directing your breath with pranayama techniques, always take time to honor your breath. Pause. Feel. Observe. Respect. Then start co-creating.

Preparing for Pranayama

Begin by taking a breath of spaciousness.
Sit beautifully.
From the inside expand, creating more space for your breath to move.
Let your pelvis be heavy on the Earth.
Through your next inhale, let your breath lift your heart taller.
Your side body, ribs, and chest rise; shoulders slide sweetly back.
There is a connection between the Individual and Universal sense of self.
Feel your breath. Allow it to move.
Honor the breath with your awareness. Receive it willingly and gratefully.
And then invite it to dance.

Expanding the Breath with Slow, Deep Breathing

This pranayama practice helps you to breathe into all parts of your lungs. This is an excellent way to become aware of your breath and experience of breathing as a multidimensional experience, as well as a helpful way to increase your breath capacity naturally.

Also, most people only use a small portion of their lungs when they are breathing without awareness. If you do not breathe deeply into the bottoms or the tops of your lungs, those tissues can start to atrophy, so this practice can be excellent for the health of your lungs.

Remember, never force. Dance with your breath. Enjoy it.

Slow, Deep Breathing

Sit beautifully and observe your natural breath for a moment, and just feel it move.

When you feel ready, start to breathe more deeply by creating more space on the inside.

Breath by breath, invite the length of your breath to extend, but be sure it stays comfortable.

Begin to direct your breath by breathing into all areas of your lungs:

Breathe deep into the bottoms of the lungs, down into your belly.

Breathe into the back body.

Breathe into the front body.

Breathe into the sides and feel your ribs expand.

Breathe into the very tops of your lungs, even feeling your breath under your collarbones and into your throat.

Exhale each breath completely, so that there is more space for the next breath.

Continue for a few minutes, and then release the technique and allow yourself to breathe naturally. Notice how you feel, and if there is any difference in your natural breath.

Ujjayi Breath

Ujjayi breath is one of the first methods of pranayama most people learn, and is used during most asana practices, as well as on its own in stillness.

Ujjayi is translated as "Victorious" (and pronounced oo-jai-ee). When you do Ujjayi breath it should be smooth and long, using the whole lungs from bottom to top.

The ocean-like sound of this breath helps your mind to focus. It is good to first practice this breathing while seated and then apply it to your yoga practice on the mat.

It should be relaxed—if you find your throat straining it is too effortful. If that is the case, release the technique almost till there is no sound, and then continue in a very subtle manner.

Another way of putting it: If your breath sounds like Darth Vader, you're overdoing it. Let it be instead like putting a seashell to your ear and listening to the sound of the ocean softly and sweetly.

Ujjayi Pranayama

Ujjayi is like an embrace of the breath, inviting the sound of waves in the ocean of breath.

Like a whisper, tone your throat around your breath softly so you begin to hear the sound of your breath come in whispering waves.

If you don't quite understand, open your mouth and whisper, "haaa." Feel the way your throat tones around that whispered sound. You can do it a few times if you'd like, then close your mouth and keep the gentle embrace in your throat as you breathe.

Breathe evenly in Ujjayi, with the inhale and exhale becoming the same length and rate.

Accept the inhale and release the exhale in a smooth and respectful flow with the Divine dance of Prana.

Breathe.

Feel.

Be.

7-7-7 Ujjayi Breath (and breath retention)

If you're familiar with Ujjayi Pranayama and would like to take it a step further, one way is to expand the space between the inhale and exhale. For instance, if you are inhaling and exhaling to a count of 7, you could sweetly (lovingly, kindly, respectfully) expand and retain the breath to a count of 7 before exhaling. (It doesn't have to be 7 either; you can do any count that is comfortable for your breath).

Once you are very comfortable with retaining the breath between the inhale and exhale, you can play with retaining the breath between the exhale and the inhale. Build up to this, as it takes deep calm and focus to pause with the breath exhaled, whereas it is somewhat easier to hold the breath when it is full. Be very respectful when retaining the breath. Don't hold your breath to the point of irritation or discomfort, instead, let it out smoothly—if you have held it for too long your breath will rush out in a hurry.

This is a beautiful practice that can lead you into the sanctuary of subtle pulsation where mind, body, heart, and spirit can soar! Try it. See what your experience is.

Nadi Shodhana

Nadi Shodhana, or Alternate Nostril Breathing, brings balance to the energetic and physical channels of the body.

The Ida (left side) and Pingala (right side) are two energetic currents and channels that swirl around the central channel, the Sushumna. When you do Nadi Shodhana, the isolated breath balances and clears the two sides, as well as helps Prana flow without restriction through the Sushumna.

To do this exercise, take the index and middle finger on your right hand and curl them into the palm. You'll use the very tip of the thumb for the right nostril, and the tips of the ring and pinky fingers together for the left nostril to block the flow of air.

Nadi Shodhana Pranayama

Pause. Feel. Honor your breath.

Then, with the chin slightly lowered in Jalandhara Bandha, lift your hand and use your fingers to close the left nostril.

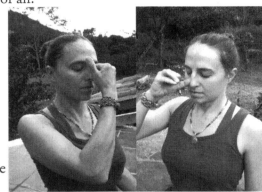

Exhale through your right nostril. Then inhale through the right nostril.

Switch, opening the left nostril and closing the right with your thumb.

Exhale, and then inhale, on the left side.

Switch to the right on the exhale, and continue.

Breathe evenly, making the breath the same count of time on exhale and inhale. Make the flow very smooth. You can also use Ujjayi breath.

After a few minutes, or when you are ready to finish, exhale completely and then allow your hand to rest on your lap.

Take some time to simply feel and breathe naturally.

Once you are very comfortable with this technique, you can retain the breath at the end of the inhale and possibly the end of the exhale, such as in the 7-7-7 Ujjayi.

Remember, it doesn't have to be a 7 count. Use what works for you.

Kapalabhati

"Light up your head!"

Kapala means "skull," while *bhati* is "light." So you can imagine this breath illuminating the inside of your head, otherwise implying that it brings great insight.

This breath uses a combination of short, powerful bursts for the exhale with passive, slightly longer inhales. Contracting the lower belly creates the powerful exhale. The inhale simply happens as the air rushes back in.

If you have a hard time isolating the low abdominals to make this action, you can make a soft fist in one hand, cup the other around it, and use your hands to assist by gently pushing into the lower belly on the exhale. Note: Kapalabhati is not recommended during pregnancy or menstruation.

During this pranayama exercise I'll instruct you to *not* use the bandhas so you can allow the lower belly to expand outward as much as comfortable on the inhale. During breath retention after the round of Kapalabhati, you can use the bandhas, and then release again if you're doing another round. If this instruction confused you, pretend you were off flying on your Dragon and didn't read it at all. Not to worry. Just breathe.

Kapalabhati Pranayama

Sit beautifully and take some time to just feel your breath move.

Inhale deeply, and then exhale fully.

Inhale deeply, down into your belly, allowing your belly to expand.

Contract your lower belly strongly to create a powerful exhale.

Allow the breath to quickly rush back in, expanding your lower belly.

Rapidly contract the lower abdominals to exhale.

Continue receiving each inhale, and powerfully exhaling, 10–30 times. (You can gradually increase this number as your practice matures.)

End with a complete exhale.

Then, take a nice deep breath.

On the next breath, inhale completely, and then hold your breath as long as comfortably possible (this breath retention is optional).

Maintain a feeling of expansion and lightness within as you retain the breath, then gently let it out and allow a few cycles of natural breath in order to notice how you feel.

You can repeat this cycle 3 times or more, with rapid bursts of exhales, followed by a deep, complete breath, another deep inhale that is held, and then some time to just feel and be.

The Space Between The Breath

As you read this, invite your posture to become more beautiful and spacious . . .

Receive your breath by simply expanding and letting it enter you more deeply and joyfully . . .

Isn't it amazing how something that subtle can feel that good?

In this short practice, you are given the opportunity to observe the space between your breaths, and how entering into that awareness can shift your state in a profound way.

The Space Between the Breath

Sit beautifully, settling into your hips and lifting up through your spine.

Take a few moments to simply observe your natural breath, noticing how your ribs expand and your heart rides upon the rise and fall of your diaphragm.

Think of your breath as a gift you receive as you open from the inside, allowing its waves of life energy to cycle through your body and being.

Once you are more in tune with the natural pulsation of your breath, begin to pay particular attention to the space between each inhale and exhale.

You don't need to direct your breath at all, but just by focusing on these gaps you may notice that they become broader and more accessible.

Continue to feel and watch the top of each inhale and the bottom of each exhale.

What effect does this have on your mind and emotions?

How does it feel physically to focus on these spaces of transition?

Ride the waves of your breath as long as you'd like, enjoying the spaces in between.

Whatever your practice of pranayama, may it be a blessing of joy and peace that leads you further into the heart where all things become one.

Integrating the Fifth Initiation

The focus and contentment you find in meditative practice is built day by day, breath by breath.

Set out time for yourself. Meditate every day.

Integrate pranayama each week, if not daily. Let this practice build slowly, with the greatest respect.

Cultivate your focus. It will take time. Allow it to take time.

Your ability to focus and find contentment is a primary access point to the love, wisdom, and power that you cultivate as a Dragon Rider.

This is a vital element if you wish to walk the path towards Mastery. The rest of the initiations in this Dragon Rider's Training build on meditation and dancing with the breath.

Remember, it's a practice—just enjoy the journey!

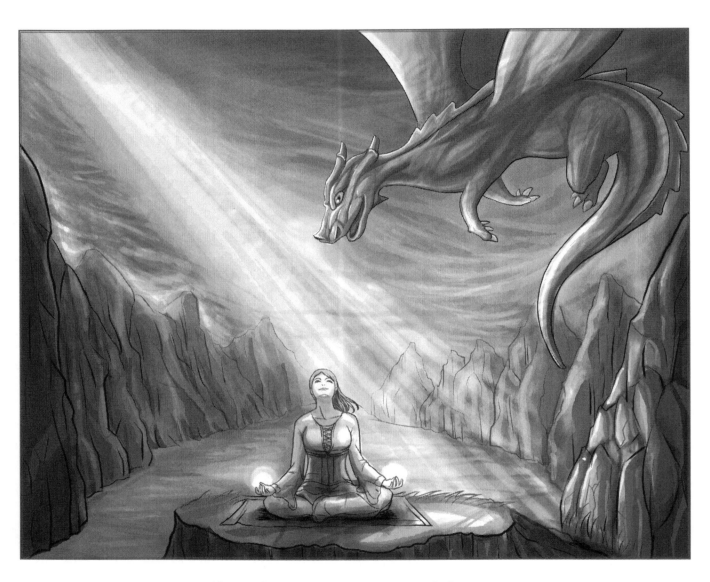

Dwell Within the Sanctuary of the Heart

Om

The Sixth Initiation:
Resonance

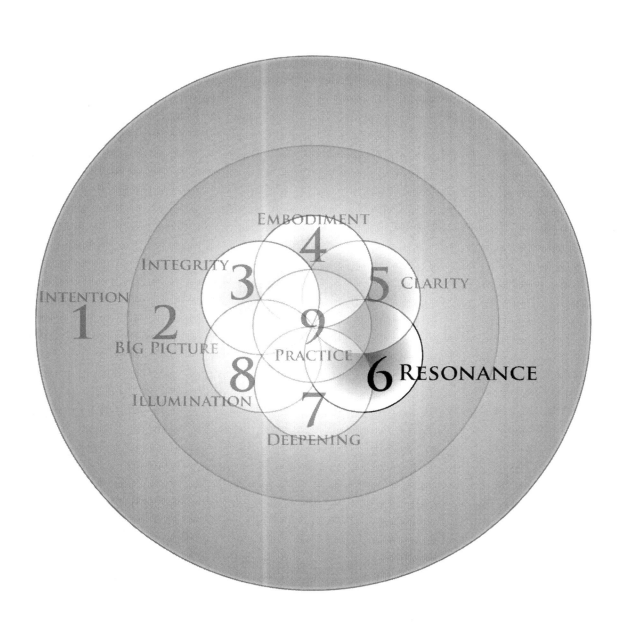

The Power of Vibration, Words, and Mantra

Remember that sound and its waves are also light,
and ripple out strongly in the manifest world in which you live.

Sound, vibration, and resonance are incredibly powerful.

The harmonics of the waves of sound can direct change, move energy, and create reality.

Let me tell you a story . . .

This book you are reading was born in the early morning hours of December 10, 2011, under the light of a full moon on the night of an eclipse.

Earlier that day, I had an Acutonics® session with my friend Karen. Acutonics uses a collection of tuning forks, as well as other instruments such as bells and tingshas, to work with the energy in your body and energy field. Acutonics is closely related to acupuncture, but the practitioner uses sound vibrations, patterns, and frequencies—rather than needles—to move the energy.

At the very end of the session, after close to an hour of energy work, Karen walked away to give me time to integrate.

I lay on the massage table, just feeling, processing, and settling.

I was also waiting for something.

And, though I didn't know what I was waiting for before it hit me, I recognized it immediately when it did.

My Dragon came to me then. A very recognizable energy *merged* with me. It was like a part of my soul was reunited with the rest of me, and it was very clearly in the form of a Dragon.

Shamanic practitioners call this kind of energetic reunion a soul retrieval. The idea is that, along the way through many lifetimes, parts of our soul get scattered and hide themselves due to traumas and other factors. According to this perspective, if you've ever felt like a part of you is missing, it could be that you're sensing a particular part of your soul that is hidden, dormant, or unable to function as part of the whole of who you are. You might feel an "emptiness," recognizing the absence of awareness from a part of your essence.

Yet when we do healing work, when we align with Nature and our inner knowing, when we move energy into a more optimal flow, we can reclaim the wholeness that is our birthright.

This was such a soul retrieval. It was so powerful Karen felt it across the room as a burst of joy.

I felt it as a surge of power, knowing, and joyful recognition of my heart.

I sang my way home after the session.

Later that night, lying in bed awake around 1:00 A.M., moonlight streaming in through the curtains, I was hit with such inspiration that I nearly jumped out of bed.

An idea had announced itself to my inner awareness and was ready to be downloaded and shared!

As I typed nonstop through the dark of the early morning, with the energies of the Eclipse enhancing the flow and vision, *Yoga for Dragon Riders* was born.

Sound and Matrika Shakti

Vibration holds power, especially when sound is charged with intent.

Sound is the bridge between thought and reality—between the unmanifested and the manifest.

Sound can carry infinite forms. For example, some music makes you feel excited and happy, some makes you want to run or drive fast, some music doesn't feel good at all and can be irritating or disturbing, and other music brings you into a state of calm and peace.

Similarly, different languages hold and express different resonances.

Think of how often the intent and feeling of a language is brought up in many of the stories we read. Think of the light, lilting language of the elves in *The Lord of the Rings* compared with the language of Mordor, which most of the characters don't dare utter.

You've probably also noticed that the oldest or original language in any story you read is generally thought of as the most powerful—as being closest to the resonance of the actual word.

In our world, Sanskrit is one such original language. *Sanskrit* means "perfected," "polished," or "refined." It is believed, by some sources, to be the world's oldest language, and most of the words used in other Indo-European languages can be connected to a root word in Sanskrit. This language is sacred in India, where mystic traditions describe it as the "language of the gods."

I am not a Sanskrit scholar, but I know that my experience has been profound when using mantras in this language.

The sounds and words of Sanskrit carry the essence of the things they describe.

When you name something in Sanskrit, you invoke the energy of it. You call to its form and pull it into reality.

For instance, when you chant *Shanti*, you are not only describing and invoking peace but entering its vibration.

When you chant *Om*, you shift your state instantly into one that is more focused, attuned to harmony, and open to the Universal current of being.

Matrika Shakti

Matrika Shakti is the power of sound and word.

It even goes beyond sound and word to all levels of conceptualization.

It signifies the importance of intent, because when you use thought, speech, and sound mindlessly, you are essentially flinging power around. Imagine a spell-caster randomly and thoughtlessly unleashing magic in one of the stories you've read. The results would be unpredictable, could be disastrous, and most likely would not get the characters where they want to go in a clear, efficient manner.

It's the same idea when we are not deliberate with our words and thoughts.

When, instead, you learn to direct your thoughts and speech with awareness, the path before you changes to reflect what you are putting out as your intent.

Matrika is an expression of the Goddess Shakti, the sentient creative power that encompasses and exists as All That Is. Matrika describes Shakti—in the process of the One becoming many—as thought, speech, and sound.

When you mis-speak, rather than thinking of the old saying, "Watch your mouth," think instead, "Watch your Matrika Shakti!"

Watch the power of your words. Be aware of the power of your thoughts.

Infuse them with intention, with meaning, with purpose.

Use Matrika Shakti with integrity and goodwill to shape how you contribute and influence the world around you, and you will go far indeed, Dragon Rider!

Entrainment and Attunement

Let's talk about the Guru Principle for a moment, because it has a lot to do with Resonance.

Guru means "weighty one."

Something that holds weight has a lot of gravity, and gravity influences the field of space-time, the realm in which we're currently residing.

Guru also means "dark and light," or "one that brings light to darkness."

The term guru often describes a great teacher or Master. If you find a teacher who has great wisdom and integrity, whose guidance you want to align with, you might consider them your guru (though you don't need to use the word guru at all if it doesn't resonate with you).

And yet, the guru is also found in all things, for everyone and everything can be a teacher.

Now that you understand the general idea of the Guru Principle, let's talk about entrainment.

Entrainment is when one thing has a stronger pulsation or gravity, causing other things to shift into its frequency.

For instance, if you have a room full of different clocks all ticking at different times, and into that room you bring a grandfather clock, you will notice something remarkable: all the other clocks will start to tick in time with the swinging of the grandfather clock's pendulum.

This is entrainment. It is when one presence is stronger than the others around it, and so envelops or influences their energies.

It was said that Buddha's field of influence was more than a mile wide. Anything within that distance was entrained with his field of peace and compassion. That's the Guru Principle in action.

Gandhi revolutionized the way the people in India and all around the world perceived injustice, slavery, and discrimination.

As did Martin Luther King, Jr.

Likewise, but on the opposite side of the moral spectrum, Hitler influenced an entire country to do unthinkable things.

In *The Lord of the Rings* by J.R.R. Tolkien, Gandalf and Aragorn are the among the weighty ones who save Middle Earth, as are the Hobbits, showing the power each of us can summon from within when we align with something of great meaning. Like saving the world.

Now, attunement is a refined and deliberate entrainment.

Attunement is a choice to consciously align with a bigger energy or purpose.

For example:

You can attune to Nature: to the pulsation of the ocean, the peace of a mountain valley, the patient wisdom of a tree . . .

The same can be done with a cause or vision—if you align yourself with a movement or purpose that you believe in, you can attune to it and add to its energy.

Sure, most people naturally felt peace and purpose from Gandhi, but those who joined his movement and attuned to his philosophy made conscious choices to do so. Once they did, they added their own power to something that changed the face of history and several countries, and then rippled out across the world.

There may be a person whose very energy and presence you want to attune to: Someone you respect so fully, and who is so skilled and wise as to be considered a principal teacher or a loved one. To attune with her (or him) you would choose to not only focus diligently on what they say

YOGA FOR DRAGON RIDERS

186

and do, but you could consciously entrain—even naturally breathing in time together. You get into their pulsation.

The key to attuning to another human being is to not lose yourself in the other. Remember who you are and follow your own heart at all times.

So, just to summarize:

Entrainment is a natural shift into the same pulsation as a powerful energy or frequency.

Attunement is consciously choosing to align with a bigger energy or influence—you make this choice and then act with skill and awareness.

Start to notice how you can use these two concepts and actions in your life.

Can you observe yourself entraining to the feeling of whatever your environment is around you?

You may freely want to give yourself over to the power of entrainment if you're somewhere that feels good , such as a forest or place of beauty in Nature. Or, you might be in a place that holds a frequency you don't actually want to entrain with.

In which case, you can attune to the vibration of your choice. You can attune to a specific tree, or you can decide to call on the resonance of light in a place of darkness.

Attune with intent. It can be silent or you can use sound, but notice if one is easier or more powerful than the other.

Try this:

In your head, think *Om Shanti, Shanti, Shanti.*
Notice how you feel.

Now, without really thinking about it, read out loud:
"Om Shanti, Shanti, Shanti."
Notice how you feel.

Now. Speak with intention. Conjure up the feeling of peace and say
"Om Shanti, Shanti, Shanti!"
Notice how you feel.

You can absolutely get the same power silently (with your thoughts) as you can with sound, however it takes a focus and a strong will to do so.

Sound as Manifestation

The last little exercise leads us perfectly to the concept of sound as manifestation.

I said before that sound bridges thought and reality.

The vibration of sound lends density and weight to something. So you take an idea—which doesn't really have much mass—and bring it into a waveform that is measurable within reality.

You can likely think of dozens of different ways you've seen this happen.

"Be careful what you wish for, it might come true!" is a classic saying that we've all heard. It's often something you hear after you've made a statement you might not actually want to come true. It is a reminder of the power of thought and word.

Prayers are often spoken. Spells are generally cast out loud. Songs are sung as expression of emotion. The concepts of plays and movies are acted out, making them happen in this world when they started as someone's idea.

And though words are written and not actually spoken when we read books, they hold power as we process them and hear the words within our minds. Through the medium of conceptualization being passed from one mind to another, Matrika Shakti holds power.

SOUND + INTENTION = POWERFUL INFLUENCE AND MANIFESTATION

Mantra

Om Gam Ganapataye Namaha.
Om Gam Ganapataye Namaha.
Om Gam Ganapataye Namaha.

Mantra is sound in repetition.

Mantras can be ancient or spontaneous. They can be sung, chanted, whispered or repeated in silence.

They can be in any language. They can be raw sound without meaning or be incredibly specific.

This is a tremendously transformational practice.

You can use mantra in meditation, giving your mind something to focus on. And you can also use it at any other time to harness your focus and invoke a specific energy.

The effects and uses of mantra are many, such as focusing the mind, instilling peace, devotional practice, protection, calming an upset child, bringing light into a place of suffering, and anything else you can think of!

When you chant, sing, or mentally repeat mantra, you have direct influence on the vibrations you experience. Realize that this is power, Dragon Rider. Whatever resonance you create ripples out to affect the world around you.

By creating a resonance of light, healing, peace, love, joy, and all that is good, you literally create these feelings in your experience. By chanting, singing, or thinking mantra, you shift into the frequency of the Divine.

Mantra is a way of participating in the resonance of the world as it is—a vibratory connection to the energy that pulsates within everything. It focuses your attention and is a form of pranayama as your breath cycles with repetition, rhythm, and resonance.

This vibratory resonance stills your mind, cleanses your emotions and brings you into a feeling of balance that reaches your soul. Mantra ultimately leads you to silence, and a pause of quiet is observed after chanting to give you the opportunity to feel the vibration and the effects and presence it has given you.

Ancient Mantras

Some mantras are very, very old.

Take *Om*, for example. It's the primordial sound. You know, "In the beginning was the Word . . . and the Word was God." Om. The word. The vibration of the Universe experiencing itself.

Om goes way back.

OM: THE GREAT, PRIMORDIAL SOUND OF WHAT IS

Om is the maha mantra— the great mantra. It is the sound that no one can quite explain fully with words.

It must be felt, consciously, to be experienced. And even then, the experience is ever deepening.

The thing about Om is that it is always there. It is simultaneously the sound from which all things came, the sound that sustains, and the sound that dissolves everything lovingly into itself.

Although this explanation may seem rather abstract, when you remember that all things are pulsation, you can think of it this way: Om is the pulsation of the eternal Universe.

You can meditate on Om alone, repeating it over and over, and attain the oneness of Universal and Individual that brings with it the most profound and complete harmony of all.

Give it a try: sit beautifully and sing Om 5 times. How do you feel?

THE GAYATRI MANTRA

The Gayatri Mantra, which is actually named for its meter (its beat), is also one of the most ancient mantras.

Om bhur buvaha suvaha

Thath savithur varenyam

Bhargo devasya dheemahi

Dhiyo yonaha prachodayath

The Gayatri Mantra inspires wisdom and contemplates the glory of light. It invokes and embraces love, radiant illumination, and Divine Grace of Universal consciousness. It is an ancient hymn that is used to bring protection and blessings to those who sing it with devotion.

Old mantras that have been traditionally sung by generations of people hold their original power as well as the collective energy of everyone who has used that mantra.

In other words, if a mantra has been repeated a great many times by a great many people, the world knows the resonance of that vibration. It is something you can attune to and feel.

Let's go over some other well-loved and often-used mantras that have ancient roots.

Om Shanti Shanti Shanti

Shanti is the vibration of peace, and this chant calls every cell of your body and aspect of your being into the domain of peace. As you chant, this peace radiates out to bring peace to the world. You may also direct it to specific places or people with your intention.

Om Gam Ganapataye Namaha

This mantra invokes the loving assistance of Ganesha, who is the Lord of Beginnings and the Remover of Obstacles. He is also the Deva of Intellect and Wisdom. This song is a celebration of a fresh cycle, a flowing life, and a welcoming of blessings.

Shri Ma Jai Ma

This mantra is in complete honoring of the Divine feminine. Ma is what you think it is: Mother. Yet it goes to the essence of mother, the goddess, the feminine Source energy that nurtures, creates, and transforms.

Om Asatoma Sadgamaya
Tomasoma Jyotir Gamaya
Mrityorma Amritam Gamaya

Here is one possible translation for this mantra: Lead us from unreal to the Real. Lead us from darkness to the Light. Lead us from the fear of death to knowingness of Immortality.

Yemaya Olodo Yemaya

This chant honors the Goddess of the Ocean. It is not Sanskrit, but African in origin.

I like to sing this with my drum, using intention to create deep healing in all the waters of the world, and to completely enter the loving flow of the current of Grace.

I sang it once with friends on a beach in Baja California, with waves from the Pacific Ocean crashing on the shore. We sang at sunset, and when the sun went down and the stars came out, it also looked like there were stars in the water and on the beach. The ocean became phosphorescent.

The Ocean heard us honor her with our song. And she was well pleased.

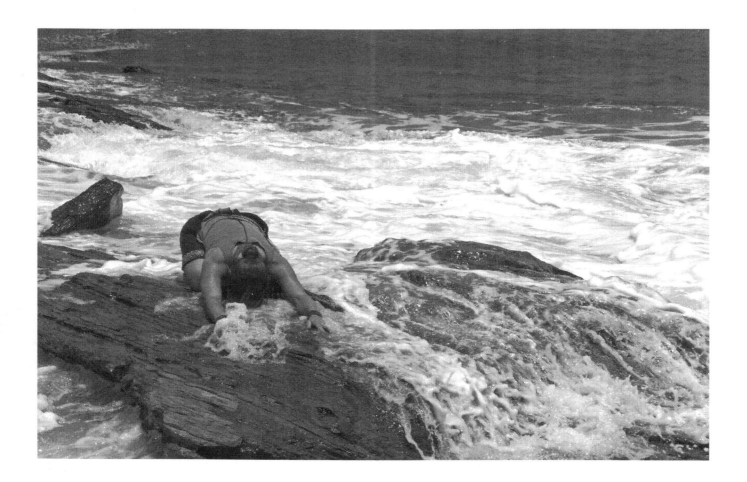

Not-So-Ancient Mantras

In addition to mantras of ancient origin, mantras can be any affirmation or repeated sound. You can create your own, or take something and make it meaningful to yourself. Then, as you repeat it, it has its beginning in your own heart and mind, and it creates a vibration attuned to you.

For example, this mantra made its appearance in my mind while I was in the heart of a forest:

Om Shri Gaia Ma, Purnatva Gaia Ma

This mantra means "Beautiful, abundant, benevolent Earth Mother, you are the fullest perfection, Divine Mother Earth." It's mostly Sanskrit, and it honors and invokes Gaia, the Earth Goddess.

Another mantra I use often is in English:

I am love and light, joy and peace.

This is a powerful affirmation that can be used as a mantra. It refocuses and aligns with a specific purpose, creating a frequency that is stronger than any other feelings such as fear or anger. It dissolves negativity and brings a shift into the purest feelings of all.

This is one of my favorites; I use it often. It is an affirmation that shifts energy immediately and focuses the mind to purpose and power:

I am pure, the purest of the pure.

I accept my power. I embrace my power. I claim my power.

For there is only light to wield!

Here's a series of affirmations that can be used as a remarkably powerful mantra:

I am love.

I am wisdom.

I am power.

I am light.

I am peace.

I am joy!

Repeat this mantra, over and over, and you will vibrate at the frequencies of love, wisdom, power, light, peace, and joy. Definitely a worthy aim!

And one more mantra that appeals to many people:

I am happy, healthy, and wealthy.

Simple, direct, perfect.

Create Your Own Mantras

You likely have your own mantras already. If not, now is a good time to begin to work with them.

You are welcome to use mantras in any language that seems right for you, though the exercise below is in Sanskrit.

Chose your mantras because of their meaning to you or what you want to align with. As you repeat a mantra you call upon its essence, you entrain with and attune to it. Notice what comes of this as you integrate the practice of mantra.

SPONTANEOUS SONG

While wandering through the forest, the city, your house, or anywhere else you happen to find yourself, you may be gifted Spontaneous Song.

If you find yourself wanting to sing, do so! You might even hear your Dragon singing along.

Give voice to the song of your heart, whether you are singing something composed by another or you find your own song, such as in the exercise below . . .

FIND YOUR SONG

You can use any of the ancient mantras already given in this Initiation with melodies that come to you. They can be sung different ways. This alters them into different mantras, but still carries much of the meaning and power of the original mantra.

You can also make up your own mantra. This is a great way to explore what calls to your heart and to let your creativity play in the realm of sacred song.

The following Sanskrit words are given with their general meanings so you can craft your own mantra.

All of the archetypes (Gods and Goddesses) can be called to invoke the things they represent. For example, if you need courage, you might chant to Durga. If you want to connect with oneness and pure goodness, Shiva. If you wish to invoke abundance and wisdom, Lakshmi. If you need to let go and transform, Kali. For new beginnings, Ganesha or Sarasvati.

WORDS FOR HONORING, INVOKING, AND CENTERING

Om – The primordial sound; a call to a bigger energy.

Namah – Awe, honor, gratitude; a bow.

Shri – Beauty, abundance, benevolence; an auspicious energy.

Jai – Glory, hail!

Ma – Divine feminine; Mother Goddess.

Namo Namah – Bowing with the whole heart; offering prayer or honor.

ARCHETYPES AND ATTRIBUTES

Shiva – Literally means "auspicious," kind, gracious; intrinsic goodness. Lord Shiva is the Divine masculine; The Auspicious One; Universal consciousness.

Shivaya – Describes and invokes Shiva.

Shakti – Divine feminine; the creative power of the Universal; the Goddess.

Ganesha – The Lord of Beginnings and the Remover of Obstacles; also the Deva of Intellect and Wisdom.

Sarasvati – Goddess of beginnings, learning, self-study, music, art, purity; the one who flows. Mother Goddess; fertility.

Lakshmi – Goddess of abundance, beauty, benevolence, prosperity, generosity and wealth on all levels; light, good fortune, fertility, wisdom, and courage.

Kali – Goddess of time, transformation, destruction, great shifting; benevolent Mother Goddess.

Durga – Supreme Warrior Goddess; self-sufficient, invincible, overcoming obstacles with ease, equanimity, and a sense of humor.

Krishna – Embodiment of God; Divine love, limitless power, wisdom and guidance, strength and surrender, skillful play and daring, music and dance.

Radha – Krishna's companion; unconditional Divine love, loyalty; surrender to God.

Ram – Embodiment of God; *Ram* literally means "joy."

Hanuman – The ultimate friend; devotion, service, play, advanced studentship, humility, superhuman powers.

Pachamama (or Gaia) – Mother Earth; nurturing; Earth Goddess.

Feel free to add to this list. You can add other Gods and Goddesses that are representative of different aspects of divinity, and any other elements you feel you'd like to include in your own sacred songs.

Compose your own mantras. Wrap them in your purpose and focus them with your intent. Let them lend power to your meditation, experience, and actions.

MANTRA

195

The Niralamba Upanishad

"The Nirālamba Upanishad ('Secret Teaching of the Supportless Shiva') is a medieval text which begins with an invocation of two interdependent verses. The first praises Nirālamba Shiva, that is to say the Omnipresence of Divine Consciousness, experienced as pure 'being, consciousness, and bliss' (saccidānanda); the second praises the Yogī who identifies with his or her own Nirālamba Shiva nature. For centuries the text fell into obscurity, but the first verse of its beautiful invocation survived in various yogic communities and eventually became known as the well loved and widely sung Anusara yoga invocation."

—Christopher Tompkins

According to Christopher Tompkins, who rediscovered the text recently, these are the two verses of the full invocation:

> **aum namah shivaya gurave saccidananda murtaye**
>
> **nishprapanchaya shantaya niralambaya tejase**
>
> **niralambam samasritya salambam vijahati yah**
>
> **sa samnyasi ca yogi ca kaivalyam padam asnute**

Christopher's English translation:

"AUM! We give praise to Shiva, the teacher, the embodiment of being, consciousness, and bliss, the changeless one who embodies quiescence, the supportless one who is the scintillating light [of the Universe]." --verse 1

"The Samnyasi, the Yogi, is one who lets go of all supports and takes refuge in the Supportless One, [through which he/she] attains the sovereign state of absolute Freedom." --verse 2.

The following in-depth investigation into the meaning of the first verse invites a new intimacy, and allows you to understand Sanskrit words more deeply. By doing so, you can glean new meaning from other mantras or apply what you've learned to your mantra practice.

You may interpret the second verse however you wish. To me, the second verse tells us that by letting go of all attachments and merging Individual with Universal, we come into limitless liberation.

The chant itself is very old and carries with it a resonance of powerful wisdom and transformation.

An Invocation of the Heart

One of the first things I tell new students in my classes is that the English translation you see below is just one possible phrasing of what these words mean.

It is most important that the mantra supports what you already believe in your heart, so feel free to shift the words some so they feel comfortable. As long as you stick to the overall meaning it's fine. And as we explore each part in more depth you will have more understanding with which to create your own translation if you wish to do so.

OM

Namah Shivaya Gurave

I offer myself to the Light, the Auspicious One,
The True Teacher within and without,

Sacchidananda Murtaye

The infinite forms of Being, Consciousness, and Bliss,

Nishprapanchaya Shantaya

Who is always present and full of peace,

Niralambaya Tejase

All That Is: the sparkling essence of illumination.

OM

Om Namah Shivaya Gurave

The very first part of the chant is a *maha* mantra, or "great" mantra. *Om Namah Shivaya* is one of the most widely used mantras in the world of yoga. It has been given to students by gurus and teachers throughout time. It is extremely effective to use in meditation and is a powerful phrase to recall when you need support.

OM, of course, is the primordial sound. It is the sound of the Universe experiencing itself. It is vibrating within everything. When you sing or chant Om, you are simply participating in something that always is.

Om contains within it all beginnings, every end, and all things in between. AUM is another way to write it. There are three parts to it: The 'Ah' sound signifies creation, or beginnings. U, or the 'oooh' sound is the sustaining factor, while 'mmmm' is the dissolution or end. So these three parts are contained in each moment, because OM is always present. The fourth aspect of OM is silence.

NAMAH is a deep honoring. It means "to bow," yet it is a bow like no other—one that comes fully from the heart. It's the awe you feel when you see great beauty like an ocean sunrise or a sparkling mountain lake. It is the gratitude within Divine love, or the wonder and miracle of a perfect starlit night.

SHIVAYA comes from the word *Shiva*, which literally means "auspicious." Shivaya describes the intrinsic goodness that exists within all things, because it is the Nature of the energy that pulses and penetrates, creates and absorbs, All That Is. Truly, at the essence of every being and every part of creation, there is this auspiciousness. That is Shiva.

OM NAMAH SHIVAYA, then can be translated in many ways, but here are some of my favorites:

- ~ I bow to Shiva—I bow to all of creation.
- ~ I bow to the goodness within myself.
- ~ I honor the goodness of my True Self.
- ~ I honor the goodness in myself and in the Universe.
- ~ May I reveal and express the highest part of my heart.
- ~ At its essence, everything is good.
- ~ I respect myself.

And you could continue along this line of meaning for quite a while.

GURAVE contains the word *guru*, which is generally translated in two distinct ways: "weighty one" and "that which brings light to darkness."

Gurave refers to the Guru Principle, which lives as us, through us, and in everyone and everything else. This is the highest self—the light at the seed of every heart. And it shows up everywhere!

> *If you know how to listen, everyone is the guru.*
>
> —Ram Dass

So, *Om Namah Shivaya Gurave* teaches these foundational principles: Consciousness is in everything. One auspicious energy pervades all, and it is constantly guiding us.

Sachidananda Murtaye

This line describes the elements that compose All That Is. The first word combines the three aspects of the energy of the Universe—Sat Chit Ananda—which we'll get into in a moment.

MURTAYE describes taking form. It derives of the word *murtie*, which can be thought of as a form, image, or manifest thing of divinity and power. So the line basically says that Sat Chit Ananda has taken form.

Sat, Chit, and Ananda are the elements which comprise the all pervading goodness referred to in Om Namah Shivaya. Let's break them down individually.

SOME WAYS TO THINK OF *SAT*

~ Being.

~ Reality. That which is real—*satya* means "truth."

~ The power to BE. Existence.

SOME DESCRIPTIONS OF *CHIT*

~ Consciousness.

~ Pure be-ing with awareness.

~ The power to know.

ATTEMPTS AT DESCRIBING *ANANDA*

~ The highest, supreme bliss.

~ Pure delight—beyond happiness.

~ The power of ecstasy itself.

Now, these three concepts could be explored for a few lifetimes, but that should give you a decent grasp on their meaning if you weren't already familiar with them. They are truly everywhere.

A more helpful approach to understanding them is to recognize them as you see them in your own life.

By melting experience, feeling, and intellectual knowing together, you enter the realm of wisdom.

Nishprapanchaya Shantaya

This line is a deep comfort to me. It affirms that this guiding goodness that is reality, consciousness, and bliss, is never absent. It is truly *always* there. We sometimes forget, but that doesn't change the fact that we *are* this energy, and it never for a moment ceases to support us.

NISHPRAPANCHAYA describes transcending limitation. In this line it is a formless quality that surrounds and penetrates all with Shantaya.

SHANTAYA is a deep, abiding peace. Shanti is peace. Shantaya is a realm of peace—an ultimate peacefulness that is complete and all pervading. Isn't that nice?

Niralambaya Tejase

This line is just as mysterious and, at the same time, revealing as the others. It further describes Shiva, or the auspicious energy that Is, as completely free and Divinely illuminated.

NIRALAMBAYA means "without support." Source has no outside support because there is nothing other than Source. It is a stable "ISness," if you will; completely free from limitation for it is All That Is.

TEJASE is a light that is always present, even if we can't see it. It is the fire of passion, the luminous Divinity that is in every heart. It is the spark of the conception of a new being, the sparkling beauty that shines out through all of creation and within the meditative realms.

Tejas is the fire that comes from the essence of the Self, the Source of life. Your Dragon knows a few things about this.

Putting It All Together

Singing this invocation is a way to connect to the deepest truth, most profound peace, and brightest light of who you are and what you are a part of. You can sing it to align with the highest intention, to remember who you really are, and to celebrate the wonder of life.

By opening your ears to hear the voices around you (if you're with others or your Dragon is singing along), or to observe the silence between the words, this listening helps you become more spacious and receptive, expanding your awareness.

By focusing on the sounds, feelings, and meaning of the Invocation, it helps you become more present. Opening your practice with this, or any mantra that calls to you, is a wonderful way to create sacred space.

Practicing mantra is an opportunity to shape your intention and powerfully shift your state of perception.

Integrating the Sixth Initiation

I hope this exploration of Matrika Shakti as the power of sound and mantra has allowed you to form a better understanding of what mantras are and how you can use them with intent.

However, it is the *practice* that will inform your experience.

Go. Practice.

Put the book down and sit for five minutes or longer, and simply repeat one mantra.

If you're new to mantra, pick a simple one, like *Om*, or *Om Shanti*.

Be still. Breathe. Chant.

Notice how you feel.

See what mantras your Dragon especially likes.

And as you go about your life, be mindful of the power of your thoughts and words. Observe the different vibrations within and around you, and how they affect you. Write your experiences in your Dragon Rider's Journal.

Notice how you entrain or attune, and what things you choose to align with.

Use words of power to shift your state, invoke light and protection, or call in the frequency of peace.

Integrate this practice and awareness into your daily life in the ways that are best for you.

The Seventh Initiation:
Deepening

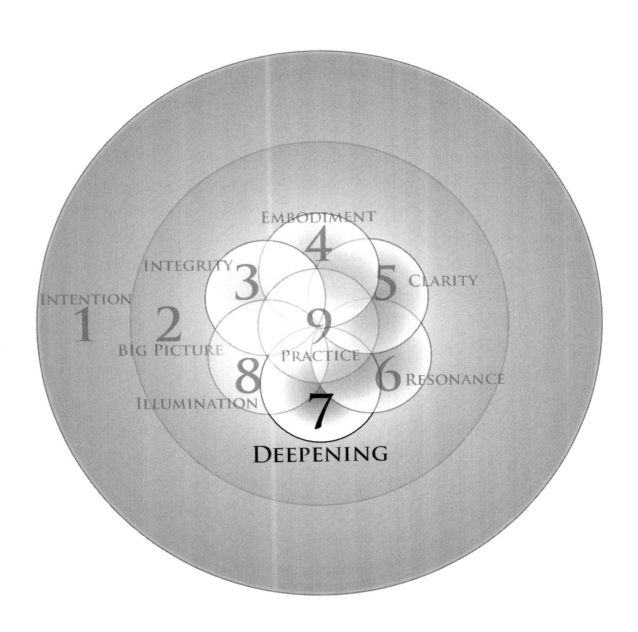

Weaving Philosophy and Reality Together

It is the ability to weave philosophy and reality together that greatly changes your perspective and experience. This wisdom, applied lovingly, is tremendously powerful. Learning to apply what you learn in yoga, in this Training Manual, and from other sources of skill and wisdom, is really what it's all about.

Doing yoga on the mat is one thing. To be a Dragon Rider you endeavor to live it, all the while diving deeper into the heart of limitless possibility. When you learn to integrate the great wisdom of sacred texts and teachings into everyday life, your experience and understanding of the Universe spirals into beauty and delight. The question is . . .

How far down the rabbit hole do you want to go?

Karma and Lila

Before we go a bit deeper into philosophy and explorations of what is possible, it is good to know of karma and lila.

Quite simply, karma is cause and effect. It is the Universal law that reflects the interconnection of all things as one thing impacts and influences another. And karma seeks balanced action. What you put out comes back to you.

As a contrast, lila is Divine play. It is freedom and limitless possibility. It can circumvent, clear, or completely ignore karma. It's the wild card, the child within, and beauty for beauty's sake.

Both of these forces affect how we experience Nature and how the world interacts with you, karma reflecting your own attitude and actions and lila adding the serendipity of spontaneous creation.

Understanding the Threads of Philosophy in the Realm of Yoga

The teachings of yoga are vast and varied, spanning time and space. It would take lifetimes to learn it all. Yet the big picture is relatively simple: seek, feel, connect, and become one with the light within.

As we approach this adventure into the richly woven tapestries of yogic philosophy, let's be clear about a few things.

1. It is important to take any philosophy offered to you in the context of what you already hold true in your own heart.
2. There are many ways to go deeper into your own beliefs and experience of Divine embodiment and consciousness.
3. We each seek a spiritual connection, and each perspective offers a myriad of ways to connect with something bigger. Find what resonates with you, and take the jewels to add to your own spiritual treasure. Your Dragon loves treasure, especially the sparkling gems of the heart!

Classical, Vedanta, and Tantra

There are three main approaches to yoga philosophy: Classical Yoga, Advaita Vedanta, and Tantra.

To explain these philosophical distinctions I'll use a lotus flower as an example.

A lotus flower grows in muddy water, and out of the muck blooms exquisite beauty.

The Classical Yoga perspective would be that the lotus must rise above the dark waters of the physical to realize the flower of enlightenment.

The Vedantic would look at it and say the mud and the flower are illusion and the only reality is the Spirit.

A Tantric view on the situation is that the muck, the root, and the flower are Divine. The mud is sublime.

Tantric philosophy is a more inclusive path, while Classical and Vedanta use turning away from some aspects of life as the means to Source.

In non-dualistic Tantra, everything is real and all is Divine. Classical views both matter and Spirit as real, though matter is inferior to Spirit. In Vedanta, only Spirit is real and matter is an illusion. Despite their differences, the ultimate goal of all three approaches is union with Source.

Yoga is not a religion. It does not ask you to change your existing beliefs or pray to a different God. The Divine spoken of in yoga is the same as the One you know in your heart. Yogic spirituality encourages you to think for yourself and find what resonates with you.

For a household yogi—one who has family, responsibilities, and participates in society—the Tantric perspective is most relevant. You don't need to meditate for years in a cave in the Himalayas to reach an enlightened state of being. As nice as it is to connect with silence and Nature in seclusion, for most of us that isn't what we choose—or it simply isn't realistic. Tantra embraces everyday life as a way to experience God.

The way that you live is your yoga.

In non-dual Tantric philosophy, everything is one. Every single, pulsating particle in the Universe—that which is in time, space, and beyond—is all Divine energy from the same Source. The manifested Universe exists so that the Divine can experience itself.

And, this all-encompassing conscious energy is intrinsically good.

You and I are expressions of Divinity. Our essence is pure goodness and love.

This invites a whole world of wonder and thought. For instance, because God is limitless, if we accept the idea that we are Divinity, then we have limitless potential.

Shiva and Shakti

In the philosophy of yoga there are many different deities. At first, this seems to be a collection of gods and goddesses that are each separate from one another, but really they are all different aspects of the One energy that is the Source of everything in existence.

The gods and goddesses that color and spice the mythology of yogic philosophy are called "archetypes." These archetypes represent characteristics of who you are and who you have the potential to be. Every single deity is a reflection of a part of you and a way of understanding yourself more completely.

Shiva and Shakti are the ultimate Divine couple. They are the God and Goddess from which all else comes. Divine Masculine and Divine Feminine, they are the first fractal-like expression of the One becoming many.

Shiva represents the power to know. He embodies the supreme, unbounded power of consciousness—the light that shines without any other Source.

Shakti is his consort. She represents the power of this consciousness. Shakti is the dynamic, creative attribute. Shiva and Shakti are always connected. The way they dance creates our world.

For example, when Shiva is water, Shakti is movement and variation—the defining aspects that make water an ocean, a river, a stream, or a bead of dew on a leaf.

Shiva is the unlimited potential of the Universe. Shakti takes that potential and artistically creates an infinite number of expressions of Divine experience. She is unbounded diversity arising from a singular power.

To connect to Shiva, be still. Imagine yourself meditating on the highest mountain; pure, tall, powerful, unrestricted and completely free in your body, mind and soul. To connect to Shakti, breathe. It is said that Shakti exhales into you when you are born, and inhales you back into her when you transition out of the physical body.

Shakti breathes you. She moves through you and pulses in every cell of your body. Shiva and Shakti are the air and the wind. They are the light and the flames of sun and fire. They are the masculine and feminine forces that balance everything in existence. Yet they are also beyond existence, present both in the manifest and the unmanifested worlds.

When you practice yoga there is an energizing element and a connection to who you are. That is the magic of yoga. It's a natural high of the purest kind.

You align yourself with Nature and the flow of energy that is the creative force in everything. The centered feeling, the power you plug into is Shiva. The dance, the art, the expression of self that shines forth in each posture and transition is Shakti.

Shiva's power flows the same in each of us; it's the one constant of life. But we all dance differently with Shakti because we creatively express ourselves as unique Individuals.

WHAT IS THE PURPOSE OF LIFE? WHY ARE WE HERE?

We are here to play, to delight, to love . . . to experience our own divinity and expand our creation. To deeply connect and know who we are, and to shine brightly.

Let's condense that even more: We are here to connect deeply with Spirit and to express fully—to realize that everything is a spark of Source.

We are all unique expressions of Source. We have free will. We have creative power.

At the same time, we are a part of something so much bigger, which also is creating. So it is helpful to think of our thoughts, words, and actions as co-creations.

You know now that the spark of Source within is Shiva, and that life is the dance between this consciousness—Shiva—and the creative energy of expression that is Shakti. You are an embodiment and living experience of these two Divine forces in loving co-creation.

By aligning with the current of Shakti, life flows gracefully. Like a ship on the ocean, open your sails to the presence of Shiva and the winds of Shakti, and you will be given energy and support in abundance.

Climb onto your Dragon and feel your wings spread wide! Shiva and Shakti are sparkling in every pulsating aspect of who you are, and all of life around you.

Jumping Tracks: Samskara and Creating New Patterns of Being

Being a Dragon Rider is about positive transformation. Rising above old patterns that no longer serve and creating new ones that do.

How is this done?

Well, in Sanskrit there is this word and idea named *samskara*.

Samskaras are deep impressions. You can think of them like tracks, grooves, or trenches that we've dug for ourselves through repetition.

What happens is these samskaras become habitual. For instance, my default reaction to disagreement in relationship used to be anger and depression. I'd slip right into the deeply dug trench of samskara that made me close down outwardly and turn my inner world into a battlefield.

Not so much fun.

It took quite a bit of work to change this, but every effort and surrender of the process was worth it.

You might recognize your own habitual patterns and reactions to life. If you have progressed far on the path of Mastery, you will have more positive samskaras and very few that do not serve. However, being human, you likely have some tendencies that you would like to change.

The good news is that you can. You can create a new pattern through awareness and vigilance, patience and loving kindness.

Here's how you do it:

When you find a pattern in yourself that does not serve, imprint a new pattern.

Create a new samskara. How would you rather respond?

You can picture it like you're digging another trench right next to the old one. The track that does not serve is muddy and slows you down. The new track is lined with sparkling crystal, and when you imprint this new pattern over and over again, you literally jump tracks.

You make a new habit for yourself. It becomes your default response, rather than a reckless reaction.

This, again, takes patience and awareness. Every time you feel yourself heading into the old pattern, deliberately choose the new one.

Practice this. Repeat it as many times as it comes up, and don't worry if it seems to take forever or if it's sometimes really hard. It is your willingness to practice this re-imprinting that creates your new experience. It will get easier over time, until you find that you spend a lot more time sliding down crystal grooves of lighthearted habits, rather than trudging through the muck of old samskaras.

Give Blessings

Here is a very high practice you can use to change how you relate to yourself and the world.

This practice is wonderfully uplifting and ripples out to touch the entire world, even though it takes very little effort on your part.

It's quite simple, actually.

Give blessings.

That's it.

When you look at someone, let your eyes bless them. When you think, let your thoughts be blessings. When you speak, let your words be blessings. When you move, let your actions bring beauty and blessings.

Here are some examples of thoughts or phrases you can use:

For the world: "May all beings be happy and free."

In Nature: "Blessings, dear tree. Thank you for your beauty and breath."

To a person: "May you be blessed. May your life be filled with love and joy."

To a child or an animal: "Blessings, little one. May your heart light up with wonder and harmony!"

There are infinite ways to formulate blessings. The idea is that you're sending out goodness and love in everything you do.

Giving blessings does two things: It shifts your own vibration into one of harmony and love, and it sends this vibration wherever you direct it—and beyond.

METTA

Metta, a Buddhist practice of loving-kindness, is very much about blessings that resonate with compassion and send out waves of love.

The following example is one I use often as an overarching blessing:

> *May all beings be happy. May all beings be free from suffering.*
> *May all beings find love, joy, and peace in their hearts and lives.*

BLESSINGS TO SHIFT SAMSKARAS

When you are learning to shift samskaras, as we just discussed, working with blessings is a very good way to do so.

For instance, if you find yourself falling into the very human thought pattern of judging others, replace the judgment with blessings.

No matter who they are—whether you agree or disagree with how they are living their lives or whether they are making choices that help or harm—you can send blessings to the people you'd otherwise judge.

"May they find happiness in their hearts. May they find peace."

By sending them blessings, you literally send the resonance of goodness to them, which is subtle, but quite effective and powerful. It doesn't mean you agree with them or what they're doing, but that you're choosing to bring something positive to the situation instead of adding more negativity.

This powerful practice ripples out indefinitely. And the more you do it, the bigger and more joyful those ripples get.

So. Make your life a blessing. Let your default thoughts become blessings.

And the world will change.

Blessings.
Brightest blessings!
Blessings of delight to you, Dragon Rider.
May this world open its mysteries and magic to you.
May you be a force of light, love, laughter, and peace.

Studying Sacred Texts

Do you get excited if you envision yourself in a library filled with books of ancient wisdom, magical worlds, and beings with super powers?

Imagine you're in just such a place. What does your library look like? What are some of the books you'd like to find there?

If you could learn about anything, what would it be? Imagine yourself finding gems of incredible knowledge. Take a tome off the shelf. Feel it. Smell it the crisp pages.

Of course, this library has many books on Dragons.

Think of all the adventures you can go on with books! It's endless, really.

Stories and poems are filled with meaning. Our imaginations delight in being engaged in the internal creation of the worlds we read.

Those books that we fantasize about in a library filled with magic and wonder, those books actually exist here in our world. Many are hidden, but for the most part they do exist.

And many are not hidden from us. We often refer to them as "sacred texts."

You can come upon incredible insight in the pages of the *Tao Te Ching* (and also the *Tao of Pooh*, by the way). You can discover depth and entire worlds of love in the words of the poet Rumi.

Your Dragon is familiar with the code of honor sacred books require: Treat these books, these sacred texts, with great respect. Even in how you place and handle them—for example, you wouldn't toss one haphazardly on the floor or use it as a coaster for your tea mug. Be humble as you consider the lineage and history of every sacred book you have the pleasure of holding in your hands.

One of the most beloved of these sacred classics is *The Bhagavad Gita*. Mahatma Gandhi read from it every day. It was beloved of Emerson and Thoreau. It is, at the very least, two thousand years old.

The following compilation is my own summary of this grand poem. It represents the essence of the wisdom given in the song of the *Gita*.

The Bhagavad Gita: A Synopsis

CHAPTER 1: *Confused on the Field of Choice*

We are invited to witness a grand meeting of conflict and contrast on the field of choice and the edge of war. Time stands still as the warrior Arjuna asks his charioteer, Krishna (God incarnate), to position him in the center of the battlefield. Arjuna sees that the similarities vastly outnumber the differences when he looks to the faces on either side—his allies and his enemies are all family, friends, and people of the world.

Caught in the narrow scope of his perspective and his own inward battle, seeing only war and grief, Arjuna throws up his hands and tells Krishna he will not participate.

CHAPTER 2: *The Sword of Clarity Points to the One*

Krishna responds to Arjuna with tough love, slices through his confusion with the sharp tool of truth and introduces the vast realm of true union through the practice of yoga.

"See beyond duality into the big picture," Krishna says. "Take refuge in the One energy that pervades all, and honor your part by living your dharma."

CHAPTER 3: *Honor the Highest Action*

Krishna explains to the open mind of Arjuna that each choice and action can be in service to the One, to the whole, and also be an example to those who are confused.

By pure authenticity to your Nature, making each act an offering to the Self, right action not only leads the Individual past the distractions of life, but also to perfect contentment and delight.

CHAPTER 4: *Rise! Fly Upon the Wings of Wisdom*

"All paths of love lead to me," says Krishna as he expands Arjuna's understanding of Divine presence and the eternal wisdom of yoga.

By surrendering attachment to the outcome of every action, you free yourself into the heart of God, who receives your offerings. Through this devoted practice, you find freedom, harmony, and wisdom.

CHAPTER 5: *Dissolving the Difference Between Action and Renunciation*

"Realize the high truth that you are ultimately not the doer," Krishna continues, "and each action becomes a movement of Shakti and an experience of the senses."

But also understand that the wise who are joined in the vast consciousness of the Universal do not cling to external pain and pleasure. They know the nurturing joy of the eternal Light within.

CHAPTER 6: *Create Harmony and See Clearly*

Krishna tutors Arjuna to find balance in all aspects of life and devote focus to meditation. This is the path to serenity.

No effort is wasted on this path. Master the mind with sincere dedication, see God in All That Is, and realize that you are ever One with God.

CHAPTER 7: *God Is All That Is*

The Essence of God is found within All That Is good and pure and also extends beyond the manifest world. It runs within the *gunas*—the three energies that make up all of the manifest world: *sattva*, *rajas*, and *tamas*. And all things both come from and dissolve into this Essence.

Of all people, few seek God with sincerity. Many worship and are rewarded, but the rare soul penetrates to fully know the perfection of God through the highest realization that "God is All That Is."

CHAPTER 8: *Enter the Eternal Om*

The Spirit of man can merge with the Eternal Spirit, leaving behind the cycles of action and life.

Focus always on the Divine, Krishna councils. Find harmony in life, live always in the Light, and at the time of the great transition call on Om, the vibration of freedom. Draw your Prana into the brow chakra and be absorbed into the Eternal.

CHAPTER 9: *The Vast, Beloved One*

Krishna tells Arjuna, "This is the high secret: though I am beyond comprehension, you may know me. Understand my boundless Nature, let every act and breath be an offering to me, and any person can through their ceaseless devotion come at last unto me—into the true Beloved."

CHAPTER 10: *The Whole Universe is Held in the Palm of the Hand of God*

"As the wise worship the whole of the Divine being they are shown the resplendent light and compassion of God," says Krishna.

Arjuna asks to hear more and listens in rapture as Krishna lovingly explains that he is All That Is great, beautiful, glorious and mighty, and yet limitlessly more than that.

CHAPTER 11: *Beyond Awe*

With reverence Arjuna asks for a vision so that he may actually *see* the vast, infinite Divine splendor in hopes of understanding more completely.

Krishna grants his wish, revealing power beyond reckoning: blazing illumination, countless faces of life, all elements and death itself. This shocks the deeply humbled Arjuna into realizing that all who he would fight on the battlefield have already been consumed by the almighty.

Then, to the frightened Arjuna's relief, the vision dissolves and Krishna appears once again in his human form.

CHAPTER 12: *The Ultimate Trust*

Krishna goes on to teach Arjuna. He explains that focusing with great love on one form of God is easier than worshiping the obscure and infinite idea of limitlessness. However, all who set their heart on the Divine reach the realm of the Self.

And if meditation and focus elude the mind, devote every action and surrender every attachment to God. Find harmony and contentment in this world through the faithful practice of love, for the deep trust of supreme surrender is rewarded by perfect peace.

CHAPTER 13: *Knowing Spirit's True Nature*

Krishna tells Arjuna the importance of seeing and understanding the elements of the world as a witness rather than becoming ensnared in drama or dragged down by hardship. He speaks about being a good person, and surrendering attachment. Through the unwavering practices of yoga that Krishna outlines, wisdom is attained.

"With great devotion," Krishna says, "follow the path that is right for you. Find God everywhere and you will see the Nature of Spirit without being imbalanced by the workings of the world around you."

CHAPTER 14: *Nature's Elemental Trinity*

Each seed of Divine form is birthed through Nature and enters the play of light (*sattva*), action (*rajas*), and darkness (*tamas*). These are the three *gunas*.

Krishna explains that those who find balance in the constantly changing elements of Nature are not attached to fire, earth, or sky and come through the pulsing current of life into limitless joy.

CHAPTER 15: *The Eternal Self*

Divine Light illuminates all, pervades all, comes to Earthly bodies and delights in the experience of the senses. It is the manifest and unmanifested, and yet is also the Beyond.

"Those who know the eternal Spirit within and without, who expand beyond earth, sky, root and leaf to truly see the Supreme," says Krishna, "their work is finished."

CHAPTER 16: *Illumination and Ignorance*

Krishna continues to share wisdom and great secrets with Arjuna:

Those who live in life-affirming ways rise into illumination and joy, but those who live in defiled ignorance create their own living hell. They get caught in cycles of delusion, grasping and lusting for what they think will slake their thirst. However, in order to reach real joy, they must break those patterns and purify them with wisdom.

CHAPTER 17: *Identity and Intent*

One's faith is reflected in life, and it is one's intention that creates or diminishes harmony.

Krishna goes even further to clarify. If one's intent is from the heart for what is Divine, there is harmony; if the intent is otherwise, there is discord.

CHAPTER 18: *The Nectar of Freedom*

By honoring your own unique experience within Nature and answering your calling you glorify God; living your truth you align with the Highest Truth. Here Krishna brings Arjuna back to honoring his dharma (duty and path in life).

Krishna tells Arjuna, and thus the reader: do what must be done as it is your work—your dharma. Yet as you walk your path in life, if you choose to give every thought, word, and action to God, you will experience complete freedom, worry will vanish, and you will be carried by the wings of immeasurable Love.

In conclusion: As you study *The Bhagavad Gita* you have the opportunity to learn—directly from Krishna—many of the deep secrets and wisdom of yoga. This text has been revered and reviewed through the ages, influencing and informing people from all walks of life. May your experience with this sacred poem—and your own interpretation of how it speaks to you—bring you much insight and joy!

The Yoga Sutras of Patanjali

Just as the *Bhagavad Gita* is required reading for any serious yogi, *The Yoga Sutras of Patanjali* shaped yoga as we know it.

Remember that great library you imagined yourself standing in as a Dragon Rider? Well, let's just say that these are two illustrious treasures in the tomes of the ages.

By contemplating these texts and coming to your own conclusions about what they mean to you, a great deal of growth can occur. In addition to seeing life from a fresh perspective, you are likely to find yourself referring to the teachings of *The Bhagavad Gita* and *The Yoga Sutras of Patanjali* to guide you in many situations. Being able to make choices and live according to a deep, internal knowing—and informed by ancient wisdom such as you find in these texts—is an integral part of being a Dragon Rider.

Studying multiple translations and commentaries of both the *Gita* and the *Sutras* is helpful in formulating your own ideas and seeing them from a wider perspective. Rather than reading only the point of view of one author and translator, you will have a much more personal understanding if you study these texts from different angles.

Below you can read my own interpretation of five key Sutras. This is through the lens of Tantra, while most commentaries on *Patanjali's Sutras* are heavily influenced by a Classical, dualistic point of view. Just to review: the Classical approach implies that the body and senses are lesser than the soul, while Tantra says that all aspects are Divine and encourages you to practice skillful refinement instead of instilling your practice with an attitude of controlling and conquering.

By studying these examples—and the Sutras included in the section on Integrity—from a Tantric perspective, you are more able to do your own exploration into these and other Sutras, shifting the voice of what you read into an expression of oneness. How? Because you are able see through the dualistic voice of a Classical commentary and instead interpret the wisdom you find with the unifying perspective of Tantra.

Developing my own ability to do this changed my relationship with the Sutras drastically, because they simply didn't call to me from the Classical viewpoint. They felt restrictive and intimidating to me at first, but when I finally saw them through the loving perspective of Tantra, the Sutras began to open like a magnificent, multidimensional lotus bloom.

Select Sutras from the Yoga Sutras of Patanjali

I.2: *yogah cittavrtti nirodhah*

Yoga is the practice of finding stillness in the pulsation of consciousness.

Ultimate union can be found by committing to the practice of refining your mind within the pulsation of consciousness. Find balance in the fluctuations and dive into the pauses, exploring and expanding the relative stillness in the Individual mind and the rocking heart of Shiva-Shakti.

I.12: *abhyasa vairagyabhyam tannirodhah*

Devoted, consistent practice—without clinging to its results—brings the fluctuations into balance.

Regular practice, over long periods of time, with devotion (*abhyasa*) must be coupled with the allowing, contented Nature of *vairagya*, giving all efforts to the Divine and having the courage and discipline to let go of attachment. When effort and ease are in perfect balance, the practice brings the practitioner to a place where the fluctuations of the mind stretch out and settle.

I.20: *shraddha vriya smrti samadhiprajna purvakah itaresam*

Practice with great faith, courage and strength, keen memory, focus, and wisdom in order to find the contentedness of spiritual rest.

These elements together create a way of life that is a constant refinement and practice, leading one to rest in the most authentic self, and therefore become deeply absorbed in the highest bliss. The elements are: *trust* that comes from devotion, *power* that comes from cultivated courage and strength, *mindfulness* that comes from applied recollection, *focus* that is built in the practice of devoted meditation, and *wisdom* deepened as knowledge and understanding and applied as experience.

II.1: *tapah svadhyaya Isvarapranidhanani kriyayogah*

The yoga of action is comprised of a fervent, transformational devotion; the study of the self and scriptures; and a constant, humble, grateful offering to God.

Light and transforming heat, known as *tapas,* purify and fuel the practice with a deeply burning, fervent desire to awaken and be in the fullest connection with Consciousness. Tapas adds an intensity to the practice that is necessary if it is to be followed through with dedication. Tapas also supplies the alchemical fire that brings about purification and clarity.

Svadhyaya (self-study) brings a contemplative attitude that instructs a deeper understanding of the self, the world, and the great wisdom that can be found in many places, including sacred texts. This level of studentship shifts the practitioner's perspective in a way that they are constantly learning and applying that knowledge integrated with their spiritual practice. The full spectrum of life becomes self study.

Finally, the entire practice of living, studying, transforming, and being is all an offering to God. For as we remember and honor the Divine in every moment, every situation becomes an opportunity to glorify the highest Self.

Every moment pulses with Spirit, and by consciously aligning with it, we are carried to the essence of bliss. These practices are conscious, deliberate choices. They are patterns we repeat until they slip into the realm of the subconscious and are ways of life. Yet each day we can choose to practice, and by doing so our actions and choices bring us to the blessed union of Individual and Universal.

II.46: *sthira sukham asanam*

The practice of asana is a balance of steadiness and freedom.

Each pose and posture we make is a dynamic harmony of steadfast discipline and sweet delight. Each serves the other, and effort must be accompanied by ease (and vice versa) in order for the practice to serve the highest good. The amount of each that is necessary can be different in every moment, yet the practice of asana always holds these two components. Additionally, the asana practice cultivates the qualities of strength and liberation, so it both asks them from the practitioner, and also offers them back in magnified capacity.

From the Dragons

When you bring together the consciousness and power of Shiva and Shakti; the fractal Nature of the Universe as the One experiences itself as Many; and all the wisdom of the *Gita*, the *Sutras*, and so many others, the idea of being a Dragon Rider makes more and more sense.

Dragon Riders transform themselves and also bring Grace to this transitioning world. What Dragon Riders bring is very needed at this time, on the edge of a great change in the world—the dissolution of one age and the dawn of the next.

When you choose to walk this path of integrity and power, of intention and deep devotion, your influence increases. You leave in your wake ripples of transformation.

You expand your ability to understand life, awaken the self, and contribute to the awakening of others.

This message is a call to action, an inspiring introduction to the intentions of Dragons and how they serve our own awakening.

A Message From The Akashic Records of the Dragons

We call to the hearts of those who are ready to make a great shift.

At first you perceive our fierceness, as is right. You feel the power and strength, you notice the beauty, Grace, and razor-sharp precision by which we bring change.

But beneath the many-layered defenses and thick skin of protection is a limitless Source of love and vast understanding. We are not reptilian as you think of them. We are warm-blooded and produce our own heat, and so we are in another category of being all together. The fire comes from the center of the soul, from the Source of all things. We know ourselves and our place in the grand design of Nature.

Our purpose is to usher in change, to bring great transformation. And we are.

We are the perfect ones to call upon to embrace and claim your power.

If you wish to wield light, and to undergo the transformation from a limited being into a limitless one, we are perfectly designed and positioned to assist.

Yes, we are fierce, but it is this fiery Nature that provides the fuel of reforming the world you know into a world of magic where all things are possible.

As with all power, your intent is paramount. Yes, the fierceness of dragons has been abused by those who would enslave us and use us for dark deeds of destruction and manipulation. That never ends well.

However, when we bond and work together with ones of great light, with those who serve the highest good and know themselves to be limitless beings of Divine Nature, we are as living fire-breathing stars, powerful beyond measure, with great purpose and inspired hearts.

When we bond with beings such as this, such as you, we help you reclaim the aspect of yourself—the part of your soul—that has hidden in the illusions of the human experience of limitation and separation.

We can merge you with your own innate powerful Nature, which is your true self and fullness of being.

And once you have reclaimed this part of who you are, together our power is joyfully infinite!

Do you wish to fly to the stars? Do you desire to shift the ways of mankind, tearing down illusions and rebuilding the world in clarity and in a mighty, honest, honorable way?

Do you want to explore dimensions of higher vibration?

Do you need us for these things? No. But we can assist and are perfectly designed and positioned to do so. We can help accomplish more when we work together, especially because the limitations on the human mind and perception are so thick and firmly established.

Like the serpent, we serve the wave of Shakti and the Divine purpose of the feminine, yet we do so with the power that has also been claimed by the masculine. We are balanced beings. And at our hearts, beyond the initial impression of fierce fire and strength, is a joy and love and drive to create peace that is fathomless.

Integrating the Seventh Initiation

Wisdom unfolds and weaves its way into your life day by day, breath by breath, cycle by cycle.

You are already a being defined by your philosophy.

May your philosophy, your perspective, and your co-participation with life be informed by light, love, and the essence of goodness.

To continue your practice, to turn the page and go even deeper, simply do this:

Take a deep breath.

Open to the part of yourself that is Divine.

Experience a knowingness, an intimacy of the Self as your self.

Breathe it.

Feel it.

Know yourself as God.

You are a unique, essential part of the Whole; a ray of light from the original Source.

You are deeply loved, and are an expression of Love embodied.

Receive each breath as a Divine gift.

Each inhale you take is the exhale of the Goddess.

When you exhale she breathes you in.

In every moment and every breath, choose to align with this Source of Light.

May you see the Divine everywhere you look.

Be grateful for every breath.

The Eighth Initiation:
Illumination!

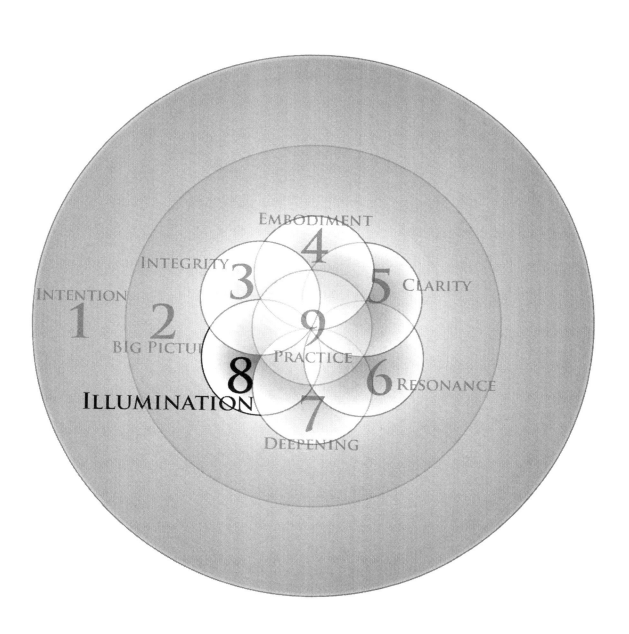

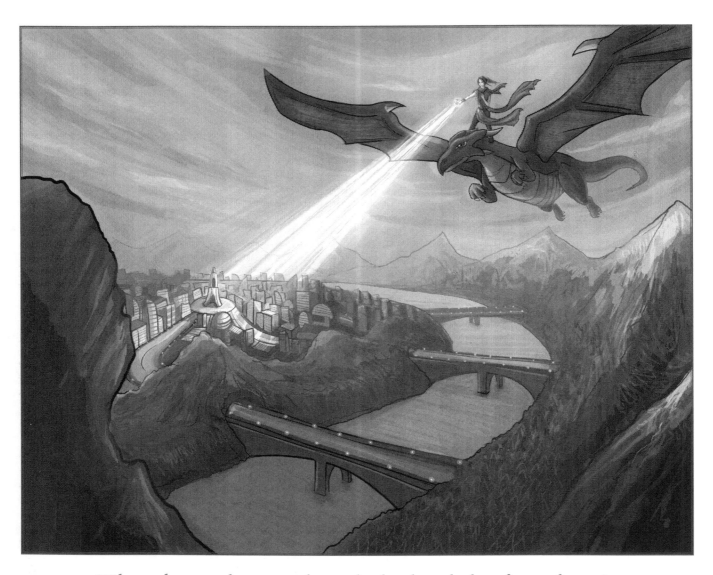

Where do you choose to shine the healing light of your heart?

Working With Light and Energy

Part of being a Dragon Rider is practicing magic that brings positive transformation and balance—wielding your power with wisdom and love.

Working with energy is a form of magic that is very real, genuine, and accessible.

Anyone can learn to work with light and energy. You simply practice being steady, sensitive, and skillful in how you visualize and shape your intention.

Energy flows where focus goes.

More and more, we are awakening to the reality that we are multifaceted beings. Although our conscious experience has been primarily focused on the physical, mental, and emotional realms, the energetic influences are profound.

Working in the realm of Light is a pathway to Mastery.

You know the feeling of being centered? You feel balanced. There is an ease and flow in the present moment. Generally this centeredness comes with a feeling of well being, harmony, health and happiness.

The following meditations, visualizations, and exercises are good ways to develop a proficiency in integrating energy awareness and intention.

You can also work with other Light Beings as Guides to increase your ability to communicate with Nature on multiple levels. Your Dragon is one of these Guides.

Know this first:

It is important to do this work from a grounded and safe place. Strength balances sensitivity.

You want to bring in only the highest light and love. Your intent is to work with pure Source energy, the essence of wisdom and healing.

Stay grounded. Every exercise includes grounding of some sort. Yoga helps you integrate your physical and energetic bodies, and you want to stay integrated. If you ever feel like the energy is too much, or you're unsteady in any way, simply re-ground yourself.

If you have a hard time visualizing you can use words or feelings to get the same effects. It is all about intent.

There is no one right way to do this, and your experience will be uniquely yours. Try different visualization approaches as they come to you. This is one of your talents as a Dragon Rider: use your imagination!

About Healing and Self-Healing

Light and energy work can be incorporated into any healing modality, conventional or otherwise. What is important is that you use intention and accept only the purest Light and energy to remove, release, and transform whatever is the root cause of dis-harmony—whatever is interfering with wellness.

If energy healing interests you, it is likely that you'll take your studies further than the techniques offered here. However, using the light visualizations, meditations, exercises and chakra balancing in this Training can be a great help and very effective in healing.

As you explore further, I encourage you to find a local practitioner with whom you resonate. When you experience sessions with him or her, you will learn much from your personal healing journey that will help you refine your own techniques. You also might find yourself drawn to study energy-healing courses.

Follow the call of your heart, and enjoy the adventure!

What it Means to Be a Multidimensional Being

As human beings, we play this game where we forget who we are. We agree to enter into the Grand Game of embodiment, and to experience the illusion of separation. And so, most people live their entire lives without realizing even a fraction of who they truly are.

You are a multidimensional being. There is so much more to you than what you may think yourself to be in your human experience.

WHAT DOES THIS MEAN?

Well, have you heard of parallel Universes? What about the Higher Self?

These are both concepts that describe other aspects of yourself that influence, but are not entirely integrated as you play this Grand Game of being human.

Think of it this way: there are many layers of you. You resonate at different frequencies on many dimensions or planes of existence, and there is an expression of you that experiences itself at those different frequencies. Part of your consciousness and energy is being human right now. At the same time, there are parts of you that vibrate at higher frequencies and have a much more comprehensive understanding of the Universe.

This may or may not be easy to imagine, so let's try it another way.

Try this: Picture many different dimensions, or planes, stacked one on top of another. These dimensions are all resonating at different frequencies, and represent different worlds. In the Third Dimension, you are experiencing yourself at a denser vibration that allows you to be physically embodied.

In each plane of existence, beings of a similar vibration live. For instance, because we humans are in relatively denser bodies, we inhabit a denser plane of existence. If you go up a level or two, there is less density and a higher frequency, so the beings there are made of different substance. In the higher realms it seems there is only light and energy.

Here's the fun part: an aspect of you resides in each level. Being multidimensional means that you are experiencing yourself on many different planes of existence at the same time.

Connecting with your higher Self is a way to tap into the Universal; the wholeness that is truly who you are, even though you're playing in the realm of illusion and the false feeling of separation right now.

Okay, think of a highly evolved being. Take an Archangel, for example. Yes, Archangels are real. And they can be in as many places at once as they want, as can many other Masters, including ones who have lived and attained Mastery as humans.

How do they do this? Well, my human mind doesn't entirely know. I'm playing in this Game of Illusion and limited capacity too. Yet there are ways I can expand my capacity and go beyond the illusion, and one of those is to conceptualize beyond the boundaries.

The basic concept of being in more than one place at a time is to send your energy there. If you are at a level of Mastery where you have complete freedom and command over your own energetic self, you can energetically be in as many places at once as you'd like.

At the same time, when you do visualizations and go for journeys in meditation, you can literally extend an energetic part of yourself into those places. You bi-locate by doing this; you are in more than one place at the same time.

Let's look at it from another angle.

You are an infinite being. The Universe is like a hologram, where every part contains the whole. The Nature of the Universe is also fractal in patterning.

And so, you are a part of a fractal-like being who exists on many frequencies, you are connected to All That Is, and the whole Universe also resides within you.

That'll blow your mind into a dance of starlight and expansion.

Let it. You don't really need to understand how it works, all you need to do is open to the idea that you are more than your human experience.

As you open to unlimited possibility, you invite an alignment and conscious connection to higher aspects of yourself. You might not realize it, but those moments of clarity and insight help you incorporate more and more of your Self—your multidimensional self.

And when you realize and accept that you are a multidimensional being, even if you're still playing in the realm of illusion, you can transcend the limiting experience of separation, and know yourself as limitless!

That's enough to make your Dragon *ROAR* in triumph!

Light Meditations
and Energy Practices

Getting Grounded and Clear

First things first. In order to keep your physical body and energetic body integrated and to set yourself up for a safe and inspired journey, you'll want to get grounded and clear.

And, yes, you can do this while riding your Dragon, in an airplane, or on water. It is an energetic connection that can be made anywhere. That said, one of the best ways to get grounded, if you're in a position to do so, is to stand in bare feet on the Earth.

For clarity's sake, it a good idea to take three deep breaths to prepare yourself before you start.

There are different ways to ground yourself. I suggest you choose one or both of the following two approaches if you don't already have your own.

Note: If you do a yoga practice on your mat, even if it's a short one, and then sit for meditation you will be more focused, clear, and aware of your body. If you're breathing and moving with intention and awareness, it tends to make you feel more grounded and balanced. If you root your femurs and stretch the tight muscles of your hips and leg muscles it's easier to sit. This is a great way to prepare for energy work and meditation.

Connecting yourself energetically to the Earth is one of the most common and powerfully stabilizing practices that you find in nearly any modality of energy work.

Grounding to the Earth:

Sit or stand in alignment. (You can also do this lying down but it can be harder to visualize and feel).

Take a few deep breaths to center yourself.

Turn your awareness to the root chakra at the base of your spine. (You can also include the chakras in the bottoms of your feet).

From your root chakra (and possibly foot chakras) extend an energetic connection down into the Earth. A good way is to think of it as a cord of light—your grounding cord.

Send it deep, straight down, way down into the very center of the Earth.

Imagine your grounding connection anchor firmly into the core of the Earth, wrapping around an illuminated crystal or anchored in a pool of light.

Then, from that limitless Source of pure, loving energy, drink light up from the center of the planet into your root chakra(s), up through your central body and out through the crown of your head. You can continue with the Pillar of Light visualization that follows, or simply use the grounding cord.

Feel your whole being fill up with light.

Feel yourself grounded, supported, nurtured, and clear: connected to the Earth.

The Pillar of Light: Into the Heart of Earth and Sky

This visualization uses intention to create a solid and strong connection between yourself, the Earth, and your Higher Self. It aligns you in a Pillar of Light, charged with power and assisted by the limitless Source of energy at the Heart of the Earth, and the Heart of the Universe.

The Pillar of Light: Into The Heart of Earth and Sky

Take a few deep breaths and align your posture beautifully.

Center yourself. Focus on your heartbeat and the natural movement of your breath.

From your root chakra and the chakras in the soles of your feet, send a connection out from your body . . . deep, deep down . . . into the very Heart of the Earth.

At the center of the Earth is a vast Source of limitless light. It is like a star—pure, loving, sentient, and powerfully healing.

Sink your roots down into this crystalline light. Wrap your roots around a brilliant crystal in that light.

Then, securely connected, drink the light back up your grounding cord, up through your roots, and into your body.

Feel the light fill you up and swirl within you.

It lights up every cell of your physical body and every level of your energetic body.

Feel the pulsation of this light as you breathe.

Now, with your own heart shining brightly, extend a stream of light energy up and out through the crown of your head.

Let this channel of energy extend all the way into the Heart of the Sky, connecting with your highest Self, which you can envision as a brilliant star!

The true Heart of the Sky is the Great Central Sun. This is different from our own sun which is a wonderful star in its own right, but the Great Central Sun is the Source of all energy, the center of all Universes.

Connect both with your highest self and the Great Central Sun at the Heart of the Sky.

Gratefully receive pure Source energy from this Universal aspect of yourself as you bring your energy and awareness back into your physical body.

As you feel the light stream in from the Earth and Sky, widen it and envision yourself surrounded by a Pillar of Light.

See this clear channel of light that shines through your physical and energetic bodies, directly into the Source of the creative power of life force at The Heart of Earth and Sky.

Establish this Pillar of Light anytime you want to connect, clear, and co-create with the powerful essence of Light!

Lighting Up The Chakras

This is a good layering exercise to enhance the Pillar of Light, drinking in the limitless Source of light from The Heart of Earth and Sky. You can also do this on its own. Use the study section on chakras later in this section to refine how you work with the them.

Lighting Up the Chakras: Meditation

Go through each chakra, from the bottom up, and light each up with the purest healing light.

See the chakra clear, balanced, and spinning happily in crystalline light.

Pulse that beautiful healing light out through the area of your body governed by that chakra.

Breathe.

Feel the shift and expansion of energy in each chakra and area of the body as you do this.

Here are the colors that correspond to each chakra as you light them up!

Root: *Red, like the clearest garnet lit from within by the sun.*
Sacral: *Orange, bright and vibrant, illuminated.*
Solar Plexus: *Golden-yellow, radiant like the sun shining from within you.*
Heart: *Emerald green, deep and pure, beaming joy and love.*
Throat: *Bright blue, spacious like a clear blue sky.*
Third Eye: *Indigo, deep as the sea. Glowing twilight resplendence.*
Crown: *Sparkling pure white light dancing with an infusion of violet.*

Golden Sphere of Protection

This exercise establishes an excellent boundary of energetic purity and strength around your personal field. It can be used alone or layered with any other visualization.

Golden Sphere of Protection

Take a deep breath.

Envision a light in your heart that shines from the limitless Source of pure loving light.

As you breathe, expand this light out through your entire body, out beyond your skin, and into a sphere or egg shape around you.

Allow the light to come from the Divine spark that fuels all of life. There is no limit to this light.

It illuminates effortlessly, creating clarity and harmony throughout your body and energy field.

Now, see the outside edge of the sphere flare up with golden light.

Take a breath and watch this golden light encase you completely in protective, joyful power.

Revisit this image any time you feel the need for protection, harmony, or healing.

You can learn to create this effect quite quickly over time as you practice. Three breaths can be enough to fully light up with pure light and golden glow of protection and nurturing.

Harmonious Pulsation

When you imagine all the cells in your body, or all the elements of the Earth, pulsating in harmony, it creates a profoundly healing, enlightening vibration.

Harmonious Pulsation

Breathe deeply and center in.

Ground and light yourself up.

Breathe and feel every part of your body and being pulsating with pure white light energy.

Now, imagine your body's cells, every single one of them, happy and content, pulsing in synchronistic time with this beautiful healing light.

Continue to breathe, allowing every aspect of yourself to pulsate in harmony, balance.

Now, if you wish, imagine all of Earth—every part of the planet and all the beings who live here—all pulsating and co-existing in harmony.

Feel peaceful and whole, powerful and clear, one with the highest love.

See this harmonious pulsation for yourself, and for everyone on the planet, and use your breath to deepen the experience. It will not only create a noticeable shift in how you feel, but ripple out to bring harmony to all parts of the Earth and even go beyond into the Universe.

Healing the Earth

By healing yourself you heal the Earth. This happens on an energetic level, and also by the simple fact that by living from a place of love and integrity you make choices that create harmony around you, and so bring balance.

You can use nearly any energy visualization that you learn for yourself to also work with energy to heal the Earth.

> *For example:*
>
> When you do the Pillar of Light for yourself, after you have connected to The Heart of Earth and Sky, bring your awareness back down to the center of the Earth.
>
> From the star of boundless, loving and powerful healing light in the Heart of the Earth, use your intent and visualize that pure, limitless light expanding out to the entire Earth.
>
> See the light grow from the center, widening concentrically out through all the layers of the Earth to the surface.
>
> See it swirl in the waters, climb high in the mountains, and even expand out to include the atmosphere and stratosphere.
>
> Send healing and loving intention into the Earth through this light, as you yourself resonate with peace, love, light, happiness, and harmony.

Again, any of the visualizations or meditations you find helpful for yourself can be applied to the Earth. Simply combine intention and visualization, and you will access the energy and light you desire.

Have fun with this! It is an incredible, worthy, and wonderfully rewarding service!

Any work you do that contributes to balancing and healing our beloved planet is deeply appreciated by Earth herself. Remember, our planet is a sentient being. May you delight in developing a relationship of awareness and co-creation with our Earth.

Ho'oponopono

Sound this out loud a few times: Ho'oponopono. Say it just like it's spelled.

Here, try this: "Ho-o-pono-pono."

Ho'oponopono is a powerful healing technique that works with love and forgiveness to shift and heal karma. It originated in Hawaii, and has been used widely to great success.

One of my favorite stories about the profound effects of Ho'oponopono is of Dr. Hew Len, a staff psychologist who worked at a hospital for high-security male patients who were criminally insane. This was a place where violence occurred on a regular basis.

Dr. Hew Len went through the files of the inmates and used Ho'oponopono for each of them individually.

The rate of violence dropped dramatically, and the people who were held there changed in very positive ways. The prison was able to release many of the inmates, or move them to other wards for nonviolent patients.

This was all documented, measured, and witnessed by the other staff at the institution.

What happened that made such a monumental change in these people who had committed crimes and led violent lives?

The energies of anger and hatred were shifted. The root causes of their imbalances were healed. And the energetic "chains" that held them down from the past offenses and traumas they had experienced were dissolved in love and forgiveness.

And that was from someone else doing the work for them!

The following exercise is expanded from the book *Zero Limits* by Joe Vitale and Dr. Hew Len, and is adapted from a meditation led by Antera.

HERE'S HOW IT WORKS:

You use intent, feeling, and these four statements. Over and over again, with a specific focus.

The statements:

>*I love you.*
>
>*I'm sorry.*
>
>*Please forgive me.*
>
>*Thank you.*

Try it for yourself, and you'll understand more clearly.

Ho'oponopono Healing Technique

You can have any specific focus as you use this technique. For this example, focus on healing yourself. Intend that you heal any harm you have ever done to yourself, on any level, in any lifetime.

Bring as much feeling as you can to each statement as you say it, and repeat it a few times. The words don't have to be exactly what you see below, but this gives you an idea of the variation you can use to bring even more feeling into it.

Remember, you're saying this to yourself, unless you're working with a different focus.

"I love you. I *love* you. I love you so much. I really love you."

"I'm sorry. I'm sorry for anything I've done to hurt you. I'm so sorry. I'm sorry, really, really sorry."

"Please forgive me. Please forgive me for everything I've done to hurt you. Please forgive me. Forgive me."

"Thank you! Thank you so much for your forgiveness! Thank you, thank you, thank you!"

Take a deep breath, notice how you feel and what emotions come up as you do this.

And then go through it one or two more times. It is a good idea to repeat this two times or more when you practice this technique. It deepens the frequency of healing and brings it about that much faster.

HEALING IN LAYERS WITH HO'OPONOPONO

A very powerful way to use Ho'oponopono is to focus on the following topics in this order:

1. Yourself

2. Everyone you have ever known (in this lifetime and all others)

3. All Human beings who have ever lived on this planet

4. Earth, the environment, and all nonhuman beings (animals, elementals, plants, etc.)

5. The cosmos (everything in the entire Universe that surrounds Earth). Ask for forgiveness from anything you've been a part of that has upset the balance.

This pretty much covers everything, eh?

While you do this practice, remember that making mistakes is part of being human, and that's okay!

Part of Ho'oponopono is taking responsibility for all that you have done, and for the part of yourself that reflects or creates the other imbalances that happen in the world.

If you remember that we are all connected, then it makes sense: If you take 100% responsibility for healing the parts of yourself that are affected by or causing disharmony, then you heal the disharmony itself.

This powerful healing technique allows you to have complete forgiveness, without judgment, from a place of unconditional love.

Talk about healing a bunch of karma quickly!

Shamans talk about walking as a Peaceful Warrior with no enemies in this world or the next.

Ho'oponopono is a great way to make peace and align yourself as an honored Dragon Rider, because by doing so you show that you understand the interconnectedness of all things, and you have made every effort to bring into balance the history of who you have been.

This technique works very effectively. You don't have to do it every day for the rest of your life (although you could if you wanted). Do it well once, and then continue with it when you feel called.

You can also choose other focuses that were not listed here, such as someone you care about, or someone who has made a mistake and needs help righting a wrong (or won't do it themselves).

Think of the healing you can create with this!

What do you want to work with first?

Write it down in your Rider's Journal (or just dive in) and go for it!

Trinities and the Three-Fold Flame

There are many Trinities. They represent wholeness and complete cycles. As humans, we bridge Earth and Sky. However we often do not have the full picture if we see only two sides or two forces. A third is necessary for the magic of entirety.

Though we won't dive into this in depth, Trinities are an excellent direction for self-study.

Some Trinities Include:

~ Earth, Sky, Human (that's you!)

~ Sun, Moon, Stars

~ Father, Son, Holy Ghost

~ Maiden, Mother, Crone

~ Saraswati, Lakshmi, Kali

~ Brahma, Vishnu, Shiva

~ Birth, Sustenance, Death (and then rebirth starts the cycle again)

And on and on they go.

Dragons represent a completeness—all aspects of the trinities embodied as one.

The Trinity of being heart-centered, empowered, and knowing who we are as multidimensional beings is thus:

LOVE. POWER. WISDOM.

If any of these attributes are in disharmony, there is imbalance that can have great consequence. However, if you have love, power and wisdom in harmony, then you not only feel whole—it goes beyond. There is an equanimity to your thoughts, words, and actions that resonates outwards on many levels and dimensions.

The following meditation is inspired by and adapted from a meditation by Omaran.

Meditation on the Three-Fold Flame

Sit beautifully and take three deep breaths to center yourself.

Send down your grounding cord and connect with the Heart of the Earth. Invite the light from there to come up and fill you. After another deep breath, send your intent upwards and connect to the Heart of the Sky. Receive the pure energy from your Higher Self into your body and awareness.

Then, as you continue to feel your breath and see yourself illuminated, focus on your heart.

From the center of your heart chakra, envision a beautiful pink flame (or light) expanding outward. As you breathe it fills your entire body, including every single cell of your physical body, as well as your emotional, mental, and energetic bodies.

This pink flame is pure Divine love.

Feel it in every part of you. Watch as it expands past the boundaries of your skin to saturate your energetic field, completely surrounding you in pink, loving light.

In your mind and heart, repeat to yourself, over and over, *I am Love.*

I am Love.

Once you truly feel this, take another deep breath. Allow the love to stay while the pink flame fades.

Then, as you breathe deeply, envision a beautiful blue light beginning in your heart. It is a brilliant sky-blue.

As you breathe, it expands. Feel it light up every part of you with the blue flame of power. See it immerse your body and expand beyond it to fill your light body.

As you feel the pulsation of this beautiful blue flame, your own Divine power, silently say, again and again, *I am Power.*

I am Power.

Do this as long as it takes to feel empowered, as Power combines with Love. When you feel ready, let the power remain while the blue flame fades.

Taking another deep breath, envision a gorgeous, bright golden-yellow light in your heart.

Breath by breath, see and feel this golden flame expand throughout your entire being, on every level, until it surrounds you completely.

As you feel the surging power of this golden light, affirm, *I am Wisdom.*

I am Wisdom.

Say it as many times as you need to fully feel it.

Feel your entire body glowing with golden light!

Then, allow the golden light to fade, and call your attention to all three elements of who you are:

Feel yourself as Love. Feel yourself as Power. Feel yourself as Wisdom.

Allow this Trinity to exist within you—as you—in perfect union.

I am a loving, powerful, wise being.

I am a powerful, wise, loving being.

I am a wise, loving, powerful being!

Know this as your truth.

Take as long as you want to integrate this, sitting with your breath and the feeling of wholeness and harmony.

Using Color

As you visualize you might see different colors or feel called to work with different colors of light.

Colors can be used in many ways and can have multiple meanings. Here are a few ideas, and you can get more in the section on chakras.

As you picture these colors, imagine them clear, scintillating, and lovingly sentient.

- **White:** Purity, clarity, truth, angelic, enlightened energy
- **Silver:** Abundance and awakening
- **Golden:** Wisdom, Divine connection and protection
- **Red:** Strength, willpower, physical and sexual energy
- **Orange:** Courage, vitality, creativity
- **Yellow:** Life energy, play, inspiration, intelligence
- **Green:** Healing, calming, nurturing, love, Nature
- **Blue:** Power, Divine Feminine, sensitivity, flow, intuition
- **Purple:** Intuition, wisdom, spirituality, visionary, magic
- **Pink:** Love, sensitivity, compassion

All of the above are healing, all are effective, but you may find that you naturally want to work with certain colors for certain purposes.

You also may be attracted to using colors that correspond to different chakras, or that are meaningful to you. Play with them and see how colors change your approach and experience.

The Chakras

Within the energetic body—the life force that animates us, that gives us vitality—there exist energy centers called chakras.

Chakras are also called wheels of light, so named because that is what they look like to people who see and envision them. They are spinning vortexes of energy within that receive and assimilate Prana. Chakras not only take in and process energy, but they can also transmit, transform, and distribute energy to other areas of the body and the energetic field.

Have you felt your heart light up with delight? Or felt your throat contract with anger or hurt? Or felt a deep clarity in the center of your mind? Or felt like the roof of your head has blown off?

At these times you're experiencing and feeling your chakras, or internal centers of energy. These are more tangible, obvious examples. However, these energy centers are always functioning at subtle levels. We are often unaware of the essential role they play in who we are as Individuals, and how we experience and relate to the world.

There are a great many chakras, and the number varies depending on what reference you use or who you talk to.

However, most people agree that there are seven main chakras that compose the foundation of the energetic body. These focal points interact with myriad energetic channels known as *nadis*, or meridians. The chakras and nadis make up the energetic body, along with the aura, or energetic field.

The thing about this energetic body is that it has a central role in your quality of life. This is becoming more widely accepted. Basically, dis-ease begins on an energetic level. If it isn't cleared and processed there, then it manifests physically. Conversely, that which has manifested physically can be cleared by balancing the energetic and emotional bodies.

By the way, "e-motion" is energy in motion. Ponder that for a moment.

If you don't let emotion flow in a balanced way, the energy can get stuck. Stuck energy simply isn't healthy.

Letting energy flow doesn't have to mean dramatic emotional release. On the contrary, emotional release can often come freely in laughter, silence, song, or breath. Tears can wash away that which hurts, keeping the body free of blockages.

HEALING, YOGA, AND CHAKRAS

When you know more about the individual chakras, it can shed light on different areas of life and how they are related to the body. Becoming more intimate in relationship with each chakra can be illuminating. When you also integrate knowledge and experience of the whole chakra system, you open to an empowering way to balance and heal yourself.

One of the great things about yoga is that you balance your chakras when you practice, whether or not you are aware of it. This is the same when you do the Pillar of Light visualization, connecting to the Earth and your Higher Self.

When you intentionally align the energetic aspect of yourself with the rest of your body, subtle and powerful transformation can occur. It is important not to force, but instead to find the harmony of effort and ease, of cleansing and releasing, opening and resting.

When you find resistance or challenges in your attitude or in your body, it is extraordinarily helpful to work through the blockages in the corresponding chakra(s) to clear the issue. Same goes for physical manifestations such as tight hips or dis-ease of any sort. Knowing the parts of the body each chakra facilitates, and recognizing each chakra's psychological functions empowers you to heal yourself.

Using the scientific art of yoga, coupled with an understanding of the chakra system, effective and profound healing can take place.

How Chakra Imbalances Affect the Body

When something is off, your body will tell you.

Of course, it is ideal to be so tuned in to the energetics of your body that you're ever harmonious and totally healthy. Realistically, however, the emotions and physical imbalances that come are the most obvious signs that things aren't quite balanced energetically. Discomfort and pain can be great motivators, helping you to direct your attention and go deep for the cause of the problem.

Chakra imbalance can swing two ways: it is either excessive or deficient. Excessiveness comes from a more obsessive reaction to an imbalance. Deficiency is caused by avoidance. In the first chakra, for example, if you are in fear and don't feel safe, you want to protect yourself and naturally put on weight. You literally thicken the barrier between you and the world. This would be excessive. However, if you were to avoid dealing with the insecurity, pretending it wasn't there, just living in the fear without addressing it, you might loose weight and become waif-like. This is deficiency.

The above example gives you an idea of the way your reaction to a problem can manifest physically. Generally, if you are experiencing dis-ease, look into where it is in the body and find the chakra related to it. If there is lots of bloating, the second chakra, ruled by the element water, may be blocked. Do some self-inquiry to find out what is at the root of it emotionally. Get the water, or energy, flowing again.

The following table, showing attributes and traits that indicate imbalances in the chakras, offers foundational information to help you better understand and work with your own energetic body. It is compiled with helpful information, much of it from Anodea Judith's book, *Wheels of Light*.

I have also included the types of yoga poses and aspects that can help balance, open, awaken, and invoke the healing powers of these incredible energy centers.

Chakra Properties and Associations

First Chakra: *Muladhara*
ROOT CHAKRA (OR BASE CHAKRA)

Color: Red

Location: Pelvic floor at the perineum

Element: Earth

Psychological Role: Survival

Identity: Physical

Imbalance: Fear

Right: To have

Attributes: Grounding, stability, desire to be in the physical world, self-preservation

Excessive Imbalance: Over possessiveness, greed, being overly protective, dullness, obesity

Deficient Imbalance: Homelessness, feeling ungrounded, playing the victim, being underweight, fearful, and unfocused

Related Areas of Body: Adrenal glands, feet, legs, bones, large intestine and colon

Aromatherapy Essences: Cedar, Cypress, Patchouli, Rosewood

Yoga Focus: Hip openers, settling, grounding, and strengthening

Second Chakra: *Svadhisthana*
SACRAL CHAKRA

Color: Orange

Location: Lower abdomen just below the navel

Element: Water

Psychological Role: Desire

Identity: Emotional

Imbalance: Guilt

Right: To feel

Attributes: Sexuality, creativity, relationship, pleasure, feeling

Excessive Imbalance: Controlling, lustful, manipulative, emotional instability, sexual addiction, obsessive tendencies

Deficient Imbalance: Co-dependency, martyrdom, being submissive, stiffness, isolation, numb or dull emotions, fear of change, lack of sexual drive

Related Areas of Body: Reproductive glands, genitals, womb, kidneys, bladder, lower back

Aromatherapy Essences: Clary Sage, Jasmine, Sandalwood, Damiana

Yoga Focus: Hip openers, flowing movement, forward bends

Third Chakra: Manipura
SOLAR PLEXUS CHAKRA

Color: Yellow

Location: Solar plexus

Element: Fire

Psychological Role: Will

Identity: Ego/Individual

Imbalance: Shame

Right: To act

Attributes: Power, self-esteem, vitality, personality

Excessive Imbalance: Self-centered, egocentric, striving, self-driven, aggressive, controlling, blaming, hyperactive

Deficient Imbalance: Low self-esteem, overly sensitive, playing the servant, weakened, feeling disliked, timid, co-dependency, lethargic

Related Areas of Body: Pancreas, adrenal glands, digestive system, spleen, liver, gall bladder

Aromatherapy Essences: Chamomile, Juniper, Vetiver, Ginger, Woodruff

Yoga Focus: Back bends, arm balances, core strength, twists; any pose that makes you feel enlivened and balanced in your power

Fourth Chakra: *Anahata*

Heart Chakra

Color: Green (also pink)

Location: Level with the heart, in the center of the chest

Element: Air

Psychological Role: Love

Identity: Social

Imbalance: Grief

Right: To love

Attributes: Peace, balanced emotions, self-acceptance, generosity, gratitude, devotion

Related Areas of Body: Thymus gland, lungs, heart, circulatory system, arms, hands

Excessive Imbalance: Inappropriate and excessive emotional expression, inadequate emotional boundaries, jealousy

Deficient Imbalance: Callousness, lack of compassion, unable to access emotions, loneliness, bitterness

Aromatherapy Essences: Rose Geranium, Rose, Clary Sage, Bergamot, Lavender

Yoga Focus: Back bends, heart-opening and chest-opening aspect of all poses, devotion to the Divine

Fifth Chakra: *Vishuddha*

Throat Chakra

Color: Bright blue

Location: Throat

Element: Sound

Psychological Role: Communication

Identity: Creative

Imbalance: Dishonesty

Right: To speak and be heard

Attributes: Creativity, self-expression, joy of song

Related Areas of Body: Thyroid, parathyroid, throat, ears, mouth, shoulders, neck

Excessive Imbalance: Willfulness, overly controlling, judgmental, hurtful in speech and thought, inability to listen

Deficient: Lacking faith, weak in will, inability to express creatively, "silent child" syndrome, weak in communication

Aromatherapy Essences: Lavender, Chamomile, Frankincense, Benzoin

Yoga Focus: Back bends, twists, also mantra (chanting), self-expression in asana, keeping the throat open on all sides (not dropping chin), spaciousness

Sixth Chakra: Ajna
THIRD EYE CHAKRA

Color: Indigo

Location: Center of the head level with the eyebrows or slightly higher

Element: Light, space

Psychological Role: Intuition

Identity: Archetypal

Imbalance: Illusion

Right: To see

Attributes: Imagination, self-reflection, psychic perception, clear seeing, wisdom

Excessive Imbalance: Overly intellectual, overly analytical, headaches, deluded, nightmares, hallucinations

Deficient Imbalance: Blurred thought process, poor memory, poor conative function, inability to recognize patterns

Related Areas of Body: Pineal gland, brow, eyes, base of skull

Aromatherapy Essences: Ylang Ylang, Rosemary, Thyme, Mugwort

Yoga Focus: Balancing poses, inversions, child's pose (forehead supported), expansion, internal focus, soft gaze

Seventh Chakra: Sahasrara

CROWN CHAKRA

Color: Violet, white

Location: Top of the head

Element: Space, pure consciousness, pure being

Psychological Role: Understanding

Identity: Universal

Imbalance: Attachment

Right: To know

Attributes: Bliss, self-knowledge, cognition, spiritual connection

Related Areas of Body: Pituitary gland, cerebral cortex, central nervous system

Aromatherapy Essences: Frankincense, Lavender, Sandalwood, Rosewood, Myrrh, Gotu Kola

Excessive Imbalance: Cult leader archetype, egomaniac, spiritual addiction

Deficient Imbalance: Lack of spiritual inspiration, apathy, spiritual confusion

Yoga Focus: Balancing poses, inversions, meditation, awareness, expansion, internal focus, stillness

How the Chakras Relate to Each Other

BECAUSE IT IS ALL INTERCONNECTED . . .

As above, so below. This time-tested saying also goes for the chakras. Although each chakra has its own function and influence and is connected to every other chakra, the chakras also mirror each other, and certain ones are directly connected:

> 1st and 7th chakras (root and crown)
>
> 2nd and 6th (sacral and third eye)
>
> 3rd and 5th (solar plexus and throat)
>
> The heart chakra is the magic mirror in the center.

For example: If you're having a hard time speaking your truth or listening when others speak their truth (5th chakra), you may also find difficulty balancing your personal power or self-esteem (3rd chakra). Another example is if you are having abdominal issues and headaches, your body is demonstrating the correlation between the 2nd and 6th chakras.

How to Balance the Chakras

FINDING HARMONY AND EASE ON EVERY LEVEL . . .

Okay, great, so it's all interrelated and now you have tools to figure out which chakra is in charge of which imbalance. What do you do about it? How do you find that ever-so-desirable sense of harmony?

Well, the first steps are awareness and intention. Become aware of what is going on, and set a clear and loving intention to heal. I say clear and loving because that is the most life-affirming approach. To be clear simplifies things and helps you process more quickly and easily. (Although the entire process may not be easy, it could certainly be worse and more confusing if your intention is not clear). Including a loving component in your intention is important, not only because love is the greatest healer, but also because you want to specify that the process be gentle.

Once you have awareness and you've set an intention, align with knowledge. Gather wisdom from great teachers of healing. Decide what approaches feel right for you. Include all parts of yourself: body, mind, and heart or spirit.

When you have intention and knowledge, it is time to put them into action—you have many choices in how to do this: Use yoga asanas or other types of movement to heal on a physical level and help move blockages from the physical and energetic bodies. Infuse your breath with your loving intention. Meditate, either with a guided audio recording, or on your own. Direct your breath and intention into the areas affected. Use affirmations that support healing and well-being in a way that is directly related to the chakras that need balancing. If appropriate, seek out a natural healer who can help you heal both energetically and physically. You also may find it necessary and helpful to process any stuck emotions with a counselor or friend.

Another way to work things out is to journal and see what guidance comes. You might simply start by writing, "Dear Dragon, what wisdom do you have for me on this topic?" Tune in with a spacious receptivity, and then see what comes.

Choose the ways that are best for you, and discover the powerful transformations that occur from working on a subtle level.

Do remember the importance of rest and relaxation. Sometimes the most appropriate practice is restorative, and settling into Savasana (lying on your back in awareness) helps to soothe the entire being.

Below is an example of how to balance the root chakra. It includes a meditation at the end.

Balancing the Root Chakra

This is where we start, at the center that organizes the energy of survival.

The Muladhara chakra, otherwise known as the root, or first chakra, facilitates the desire and ability to be here in the physical world. Its energy is mainly concerned with survival, physical well-being, and feeling at home.

Do you notice the ungrounded feeling that comes when you don't feel safe? When you worry about basic needs, or when there is a feeling of scarcity financially or otherwise, you tend to feel anxiety and fear. On the other hand, when you have all you need, there is a natural comfort and peace. The wisdom offered by yogic philosophy is that you really do have all you need, even when you perceive otherwise.

It is important to start with the root chakra when working with these energy centers, because this is the most fundamental, foundational chakra. In life, if you don't have enough to eat, you aren't very focused on creative expression because there is a more primal need that must be met. When the energy of the Muladhara is balanced, it supports and allows for harmony in all other aspects of the self.

When anxiety comes, or when you've dealt with a trauma that has resulted in fear, or when you feel ungrounded and not at home, there are simple things you can do to balance the root chakra and find peace again.

One very helpful choice is to make a direct connection to the Earth. Get outside, enjoy the natural beauty that is offered so freely, hug a tree—do whatever feels appropriate to you as a way of affirming your rightful place in this natural world. A good way to attune with the natural environment wherever you are, especially when you're traveling, is to take a handful of soil and smell it. Engage your surroundings by using your senses.

The key to finding harmony in the first chakra is to trust. Settle. Be cradled by the energy that supports you, be cradled by the Earth, be cradled by your beliefs. Be cradled in the love from your Dragon.

Keep telling yourself the truth: *I am worthy of being loved. I am supported. I am safe.*

Meditation for the Root Chakra: Transform with Grace and Support

Sit comfortably.

Widen your sit bones, either by using your hands or by leaning forward and pushing your inner thighs back and apart. Doing this widens your pelvic floor and assists your body in feeling supported.

Settle into your hips and legs. Allow your pelvis to become weighty.

Keeping your pelvis heavy, rise up with your breath so your spine is tall, your heart is lifted, and your throat is open.

With each inhale, keep your pelvis descending, your eyes soft and heavy.

With each exhale, maintain a settled feeling in your pelvis, while staying tall through your spine.

Breathe like this for a little while, becoming more grounded and at ease with each breath.

Tell yourself the deepest truth:

I am grounded in the Earth.

I am safe. I am at home. I'm okay.

I have what I need to be healed.

Allow the energy flow of your pelvis to continue to root into the nurturing Earth beneath you. Enjoy the content, peaceful feeling that comes with being balanced and grounded both energetically and physically.

Chakras and Energy Work

Clearing, balancing, and aligning the chakras brings immense healing and empowerment.

You also can focus on specific chakras to enhance a certain quality or feeling.

For example:

- ~ Muladhara (root) for strength
- ~ Svadhisthana (sacral) for creative flow
- ~ Manipura (solar plexus) for power
- ~ Anahata (heart) for love
- ~ Vishuddha (throat) for clear communication
- ~ Ajna (third eye) for insight
- ~ Sahasrara for Divine connection

You also can use the previous Root Chakra Meditation example combined with the information in the chakra table given earlier, and intuitively devise meditations and visualizations that help you practice aligning with light in specific ways for each chakra.

You may or may not feel called to work intricately with the chakras at this time, and that's fine. You might just light them up briefly in meditation such as described in the Pillar of Light practice. You may find that you dive in deep later in your journey.

It is, however, important to get to know the chakras and their influence in your life and energy, since these spinning vortexes of Prana have a lot to do with healing, balance, and powerful flow of energy.

From The Akashic Records

Wisdom from the Library of Light

Learning to read the Akashic Records or using another method to connect directly and telepathically to different sources of Divine expression can be undeniably life changing and indeterminately helpful.

If you want to learn, my suggestion is to find someone who teaches how to read the Akashic Records or another method to access Source information. There are many ways to do this. I learned first to read the Akashic Records, and my experiences and intuitive abilities have expanded from there with the Records as my foundation and guiding technique.

The following readings are some of the most beautiful, impactful, and revealing messages I've received while reading the Akashic Records or otherwise connected directly with the voice and influence of Masters and Light Beings.

Often there are several contributing voices of intelligence coming through, communicating with incredible feeling as well as words and images. The natural location, context or even an element of timing—dawn, solstice, full moon eclipse, etc.—often acts as part of the council.

That's actually a really good way to think about this: I'm communicating with a council of Masters.

These beings come from a place of incredible love and light. They show us how astoundingly sentient the Universe is. On every level.

Notice, as you read the passages, how the voices and communications differ—the words and style of speaking is very different from one message to another. Consider how many ways there are to connect to Source and receive communication.

Know this, Dragon Rider: These teachings are not often shared. Realize the privilege of reading these words. They come from wise, powerful, highly evolved beings and from the direct Source of all wisdom, the consciousness of God. That said, they are still coming through the lens of my own perspective.

Therefore, seek out the wisdom that is here for you. You will feel it and know it.

You'll also notice the themes of love and joy, power and play, humility and Grace in transition.

On Dignified Humility

From my own Guides . . .

Humility allows you to serve your purpose here. Being dignified in humility is part of that purpose. It brings you to God, allows you to rest in the palms of God, be cradled knowingly in God's love, and act with willful conscious awareness bolstered by the power of Grace.

Humility brings you closer to your heart Source. Humility puts you in touch with who you truly are.

From the Akashic Records of the Caribbean Sea

Context: I was sitting on a beach in the Caribbean, and connected to the sea herself, as well as Christ Consciousness. This message came just after I'd charged some small quartz crystals with intention of love and healing and tossed them into the ocean.

The Caribbean Sea

Love and love and love rolling pulsing evolving; reclaiming and offering.

Absolute power is also absolute beauty, and they are limitless in how they may be expressed.

This ocean is one of love and leaderless exploration. It is for the heart to guide.

Shakti lives and plays here in all her forms, yet if you choose to attune to love, to trust to Divine protection, to be very present, treasure abounds, and you will be guided to it.

This frequency exists strongly here, but is accessible anywhere. Especially when you have bathed in my waters and offered your love.

And the gift of the crystal is graciously accepted, though small, it is a worthy gift for it carries a strong will to heal, to make right, to love into harmony the imbalances that have occurred.

Simply enjoy yourself and attune to the rhythm of love. Attune to the power. Attune to the vast possibilities so that you are more able to open to treasure in all areas of your life.

From the Akashic Records of Mother Earth

Context: I connected with the consciousness of the planet. Here are the questions I asked and the responses I received.

My initial feelings: even temper, contentedness, steadiness, soft depth . . .

> Me (my question to Mother Earth): What do you need most from us as humans right now?

Mother Earth

LOVE. Love yourselves. Love each other. You will naturally be more kind in all endeavors because of this.

Realize the elements that support you are sacred. Teach respect and cherish the resources of the land.

Play. This is your playground. There is entirely enough working going on. PLAY! Through freedom and creativity, through dance and games, through laughter and tears you discover who you are.

Live freely. Be childlike.

> Me: What about peace?

What about it? You all know in your hearts its importance. There are very simple ways to create it. Do so.

I am not concerned too much about what you choose. I will keep changing, living, growing, playing. It is up to you if you want to continue to live here too. The Earth will breathe and shift in many ways. Life will continue.

Dear one, you are so special to me. I love you more than you even feel in your heart. Let our lives be intertwined in the best possible way, for the highest good of all, in the name of love, light and lila! [Divine play]

From the Akashic Records of Shiva Nataraj

Context: Wow. This was my first brush with such a powerful conscious connection with a direct and very charged expression of God. I had been in my Records earlier that day and was told to connect with Shiva. This message came as I was sitting at the feet of a Shiva Nataraj murti (statue) that was towering over me.

Note: I don't really suggest initiating an energetic connection of this degree of power unless you have a strong, grounded, guided readiness.

My initial feelings: Sound, light, and odor are enhanced. There is a deep contentment and a strong inner pulsation . . .

Shiva Nataraj

Anything is possible. The turn of my wrist and foot in the dance are whole worlds of life and light. I am here to not only show you the joy, but to bring you into it. Every detail is auspicious if used in a life affirming way.

You are Divine! When you reach wildly and gracefully into the mystery I am always there to dance with you. I will lead you further into the heart of yourself. Always dance with me even in the stillness of reflection.

Notice that I do not kill demons, I use them as **Earth: transmute the energy of confusion and darkness into the foundation of light.**

[Note: the last part of this sentence was strongly emphasized with energy, indicating that the whole sentence holds multiple pieces of significance.]

Just as the smallest move of my finger creates ripples and vibration through time and space, so do your thoughts. Use this knowledge well. Refine, without judgment, as you learn to dance with more freedom, more love, more Grace.

Wild movement is contained in stillness. Wild sound is contained in silence.

Play with this. Enjoy it. I love you. I am always in your heart dancing with you. The more you remember me, the more beautiful and majestic the dance.

Together we make magic. Feel the rhythm—contribute your delightful Divine song. Let others rejoice in your dance and they will find their own.

Celebrate YOU. And as such be with me.

Always. All ways.

Just closed Records. Whoa!!! Pulsing, rocking, wildness! I feel like I'm going to burst with loving, dancing energy!

Into the Akashic Records of The Bhagavad Gita

Context: While studying this ancient sacred text I decided to dive into its Records and see what I felt and heard. Halfway through, something unexpected happened and another voice was added.

The Bhagavad Gita

Rejoice! You come to the heart of love and wisdom, to the path of true royalty. This is the way to deepest delight and sparkling, bubbling joy! You already walk this path, yet this text so dearly wants to lead you more completely into the mystery, diving down the rabbit holes of Grace.

Rejoice! For your heart knows truth when you read these words of God, and even more you have the skill to interpret for yourself and see the glimmering pieces which are most relevant for you. This text is ever unfolding. Allow it to be so for you—an unending gift of love.

Rejoice, dear child of Goddess laughter, for you have reached the warrior's tenderness. You walk in a realm of magic and limitless wonder—here you will find the keys to all you desire. Open without hindrance to what is given and the purest star-birthing light is yours.

Rejoice, dear one. Rejoice.

18:46–47 ~ This is the golden key. Do your own work. Live your dharma. Be your Divine self and offer all your actions to the Divine. By honoring your own unique experience and calling you glorify God. By being true to yourself you align with the Highest Truth. By taking joy in the giving and being receptive without clinging, worry vanishes and you are carried by the wings of immeasurable love (Shiva), fueled by imperishable energy (Shakti).

See life like the Gita. In each moment time offers you lessons and joys, yet each of these petals leads to the jewel heart which is revealed more completely in some instances than others. Then, through your practice, you will begin to see the jewel in each petal (each aspect of life), and as you taste and touch and see and hear and smell each aspect of the growing rose vine of life you will thrill at the grand realization that pulses in you and all around you: "ANANDA" it sings, "I am that I am." All is God. All is Goddess. All is within you, and you are beyond it all.

You are a warrior priestess, serving in your star-born work. Allow your work to be an open offering gliding from your hands and heart. As you put it out into the world it becomes God's work and there is no need to grasp at it. Simply keep receiving of the Source and offering of the highest skill and love. This is healing, this unrestricted flow— this is the way of Nature. This is how suffering melts in the sweetness of purity.

Me: Thought—go into the records of Krishna from here?

Yes, yes! Dive deeper into the Self. Invite Krishna to the party.

[Invoking Krishna *within* the Delight of the Bhagavad Gita—feeling completely held and surrounded in love.]

Krishna

Ah! Come to me. Let me rock you in the arms of delight, let us dance in the heart of infinity and melt upon the poet's tongue. Let me surge in your veins and take you to the highest light. Yes, this pulsing joy is ours together. Let me breathe you in the nectar of bliss.

Asana is the ability of holding the body in the dance of ecstasy.

Stay with me. Be with me. I will take you to the highest bliss and you need never come down. Just stay with me, breathe with me, let all life be in deep connection with me. Be not clouded by ideas of separation, but let them simplify, clarify this infinite world.

It is I, always I. See layers of awareness and conscious play. Lila, dear one. You are lila, and delight ripples through the Universe and beyond because of You as we are I – together, us.

You and I.

Come into the oneness and dwell here. Here all crystals sing, all stars dance cloud colored marvels of creation. Here anything is, and everything can be.

Me: What do I do with dark/worried thoughts?

Give them to me. Give it all to me. You are off the hook, love, when you just offer it all to me. You choose complete freedom when you surrender all your actions, words, and thoughts to me. In doing this you are completely free.

Yes, there is delight here. Be the jewel heart. See the jewel heart. See all from the seat of the jewel heart and allow the jewel light to illuminate your world.

Allow your life, allow yourself to be an experience of God.

Om Krishna Prema Om Krishna Prema Om Krishna Prema

You can always access me, even this powerfully. Just ask. Call to me, your beloved Krishna. Krishna Beloved. Om Krishna Prema. I am here in the jewel seat of your heart, lighting your world and illuminating your being. We can always be in the poet's nectar, beloved. Let us dwell together here in the lens of love.

From the Ascended Master Mary

Context: To get closer to this being who has been beloved of so many and showed up as my guide, I accessed her via the Akashic Records. Here is what she had to share:

Mary

Welcome to the frequency of love. You can access it at any time, in any position, and even in any state of mind. Love is the Master Frequency, and you have moved into the higher realms of frequency, thus you are an Earth Keeper of the vibration of love.

This is a high honor and gift, it is a high choice, for it is one you have made on many levels, over and over again to strengthen and ensure you reached this place.

You have entered the Master's Matrix—one of great, unwavering, limitless love and light.

Because you have consciously chosen to be love, your ability to use its power and Grace is so much more complete and accessible.

Love is who you are now. It radiates from you, pulsing as you and your thoughts, words, and actions. You are a being of love, and therefore simply by being you bring more love to the planet and to the collective existence.

Any time you chose to align with love in your experience in time-space, you amplify love even more. All service that you do from a loving intention is given even more light and power. All service. Including that which you do for yourself. Especially that!

When you see the essence of God in each thing, when you see beauty and seek out the good and the gift—that which you see is Love. The essence is love, for within love exists both awakening and delight. Within love exists joy and peace.

This is the Master Frequency. Use it well.

Breathe. Be Love. See beauty. Be love.

And as you are love you share love, and the frequency of love strengthens.

Just as the frequency of Earth increases exponentially, so do frequencies of light multiply in ever-expanded ways. This is how you and other lightworkers are truly changing Earth's destiny and opening a whole new and glorious playground of possibility.

Enjoy. Love. You are doing very well.

Connect with me through beauty and love. When you think, chant, say or sing "Ma," let it be Divine Mother's heart-arms that hold you. All the Goddesses are different strand-rays of the love-light-web of Divine Mother.

Beauty. Love. Ma.

Simply enter awareness of love and you are with me.

Connections

We all have unseen Guides. Masters, teachers, loved ones. Angels. Light Beings.

Your Guides help you understand yourself and life around you. They help you to carry out your purpose.

There are many levels of existence. We are multi-dimensional beings and there are others contributing to our lives, as well as to the greater picture of all of Earth.

You can use intuitive exercises to connect with your Higher Self and Guides. Such methods include meditation, journaling, going into the Akashic Records, shamanic journeying, and simply by becoming sensitive and attuned.

Dreams are also brimming with symbols and things to teach you. Just read the metaphors, rather than getting caught in the weird dramas or scenarios that are presented. Write down your dreams and ask for the Big Picture messages to come to your awareness. Look up Lucid Dreaming to understand more about dreams and what you can do when you are actually aware that you're dreaming.

Your Dragon, of course, is one of your Guides. Take time in meditation and invite a deeper connection so you can be informed more fully and flowingly by this wise, loving, powerful being who has chosen to befriend YOU!

Here are some of the ways Guides show up:

There are many books and websites that can help you learn more about specific members of the following groups. This outline just gives you an overview of some possible beings that may be helping you already or show up along your adventure in life.

Power Animals

Most people have one or more animals they identify with or find significant. Know yours by seeing what shows up for you in meditation, dreamtime, and intuitive journeys, as well as those you are naturally attracted to and feel a connection with.

There are a wide variety of books and even power animal card sets that can help you attune with and access the different attributes of power animals. This is a wonderful way to receive guidance as well as establish a stronger connection with Nature.

Archangels

Archangels are powerful Light Beings who are advanced expressions of Divine Consciousness. Each of the Archangels has a specialty, or focused purpose.

Here's a brief list of some of the Archangels. You would do well to consider looking into these beings further as they do profound work and assist any who call to them.

Archangel Michael – Name means "He who is like God."

Guidance, flawless protection, strength and justice.

Archangel Raphael – Name means "God Heals."

Powerful healing, comfort, guidance in finding harmony.

Archangel Gabriel – Name means "God is my Strength."

Nurturing, arts and communication, strength, the messenger.

Archangel Uriel – Name means "Flame of God" or "God is Light."

Inspiration, lights the way, provides assistance in great change.

Archangel Ariel – Name means "Lioness of God."

Guardianship of Mother Earth, caretaker of Nature and the realm of the elementals.

Archangel Metatron – "He who is very close to God" or "Angel of the Presence."

Unity, truth, leader and guide of children, will help you claim and embrace your own power.

Archetypes

The archetypes, Gods, Goddesses and deities are all ancestors and Guides of humans, Dragon Riders and yogis alike.

The strange thing about all the Gods and Goddesses of Hindu and yogic philosophy is that when you get down to the essence of the belief you'll find only one all-encompassing energy; a singular Divinity that creates everything out of itself.

But the role the Gods and Goddesses serve as archetypes is to help us humans understand the attributes of Divinity within ourselves.

Every deity is an archetype, and each archetype resides within us. Here is the same list provided in the Sixth Initiation, Resonance, with some of the main Gods and Goddesses.

> *Shiva* – Literally means "auspicious," kind, gracious; intrinsic goodness. Lord Shiva is the Divine masculine; The Auspicious One; Universal consciousness.

> *Shivaya* – Describes and invokes Shiva.

> *Shakti* – Divine feminine; the creative power of the Universal; the Goddess.

> *Ganesha* – The Lord of Beginnings and the Remover of Obstacles; also the Deva of Intellect and Wisdom.

Sarasvati – Goddess of beginnings, learning, self-study, music, art, purity; the one who flows. Mother Goddess; fertility.

Lakshmi – Goddess of abundance, beauty, benevolence, prosperity, generosity and wealth on all levels; light, good fortune, fertility, wisdom, and courage.

Kali – Goddess of time, transformation, destruction, great shifting; benevolent Mother Goddess.

Durga – Supreme Warrior Goddess; self-sufficient, invincible, overcoming obstacles with ease, equanimity, and a sense of humor.

Krishna – Embodiment of God; Divine love, limitless power, wisdom and guidance, strength and surrender, skillful play and daring, music and dance.

Radha – Krishna's companion; unconditional Divine love, loyalty; surrender to God.

Ram – Embodiment of God; *Ram* literally means "joy."

Hanuman – The ultimate friend; devotion, service, play, advanced studentship, humility, superhuman powers.

Pachamama (or Gaia) – Mother Earth; nurturing; Earth Goddess.

Masters

There are a great many Ascended Masters who devote themselves to helping us on Earth. These Masters include those we call Gods and Goddesses.

Some of these Masters include:

Buddha

Christ

St. Germain

Isis

Portia

Goddess Liberty

Goddess Justice

Gaia

Mary

Melchizedek (also an Archangel)

Kuthumi

These are only a very few. There are many, many Masters.

You can learn about them and also connect with them through the clarity and purity of your intent.

To do this: Ground yourself, light yourself up so only 100% pure light can enter your field (the Pillar of Light meditation is good for this), and then intend to connect to a specific Master. It can be helpful to state your intention and the Master's name out loud, and you may find that it helps to write as you receive information. You can ask a question or simply see what comes. Be clear, yet spacious. Receive whatever energy or messages the Master gives you.

They particularly enjoy helping those who are upon the path of Mastery.

Crystals

Crystals can provide many different levels of assistance, from direct communication to the ability to bring specific frequencies of attunement.

Crystals are very sentient and can be both Guides and tools that direct and amplify energy. They are also excellent for transforming negative energy into light.

I recommend that you explore this realm of vibration and beauty on your own, and see what you find.

FROM THE AKASHIC RECORDS OF THE MINERAL KINGDOM

Initial feelings: A soft, high vibration. Feels good, very light. Eyesight more clear when looking at crystals. Floaty. Slow motion feeling. Presence. Awareness. Solemn, playful wisdom. Clear laughter!

> Me: What can I do to enhance knowledge and abilities with crystals?

Tune In. Feel the heartbeat of vibration. [Feels very peaceful.]

> Me: What is the work that the Mineral Kingdom is doing here on Earth?

VAST support. Knowledge and wisdom keepers, communicators of subtle frequencies and subtle creation. Holders of energy, transmuters of energy. Healers. Conductors of the matrix of light, structure of the matrix of light. Balancers of layers of life/existence. Individual work.

Solid reminder to believe in magic and a portal into the expansive world of light. Reminder of your own greatness and of LOVE that is tangible in its intangibility.

The sparkly gifts you so love are little friends of brightness, lightworkers in their own ways. Let them do their subtle work in every layer of your awareness—even those you are not yet aware of.

Sacred Geometry is the structure of everything. Minerals and crystals exist and work within the structure. The more aware you are of the structure the easier it is for info to be received from source to source. We are essence of God that is malleable and mutable, refined and re-cognized.

Crystals and other minerals are like nervous system of the Earth. You are attracted to tapping into the signals of this grand matrix.

ME: Any other message?

Respect. Fearlessness. You are always surrounded by this matrix of light—use it to bolster your own efforts of ascension and teaching. Allow the Mineral Kingdom to lend power to your efforts.

Be deeply peaceful—learn the fathomless depth of peace from us. Learn the VASTness of the light with us. We are tools AND wielders of light. Not only to be used but we also have our own consciousness. Respect us and use us fearlessly!

Nature, Elements, and Trees

Communicating with and deeply feeling connected to Nature brings incredible joy.

You can connect with and receive messages from all manner of elements, places, and living beings. Here are some ideas:

Oceans

Mountains

Forests

Trees

Plants

Lakes

Rivers

The Sky

Inner Earth

Sacred Places and Ruins

Every aspect of Nature is sentient.

You may connect with the great intelligence of the Ocean, though there are also countless beings within it. You may converse with one specific tree and yet feel the whole forest.

Develop your relationship with Nature as you relate to everything around you. Feel the intimate interconnectedness you share with the natural world. Learn from the consciousness that weaves through water and breathes all beings.

From the Akashic Records of the Plant Kingdom

Initial feelings: Vibrancy. Many frequencies. Soft . . . gentle . . . ease. Simple delight in breathing and the cycles. Rainbows of light. Heart space, vast, peaceful, subtle yet very conscious. Humble delight in creative expression. Interconnectedness of all elements.

Hello dear one. We love you too. [Sweeping love washes over me and through me.] You have come to experience connection. We give you this. We nourish you in the way you so long to be nourished.

The elder deep hearts of trees reflect your own strength and being. You embrace us to embrace the love of God in one of the most gentle of manifestations.

We remind you of limitlessness, of the patterns that weave throughout that-which-is. We bring, give, and anchor light for the planet and humanity. We bring breath—this is so under appreciated—but the subtleties move into deeper layers of your consciousness. The influence is there.

The reality of our support and the beauty that is most helpful to remind you who you are is ever present. We are ever present. There is no such thing as devastation. We re-grow. We offer and teach replenishment.

We breathe love. We help open and expand your ideas of what-can-be through our infinite diversity.

We invite you to sway in the wind with us. We whisper wisdom and our spirits invite you to play. You can tune into our vibrations and receive a spectrum of knowledge and guidance.

We aid in healing in more ways than you realize. Taste our essence—the essence we share, by our presence, foods, many uses and many beauties.

Let us invoke wonder in you. Let us dance with you, dance upon us (grass), around us, and within us (forest). Let us tickle your skin and delight your taste. Let us be with you, in your life as part of your family.

When you take us into your heart, as you have done, with such love and reverence, we are more able to help you realize your intentions and purposes.

We teach you to be.

Delight in our colors. Feel our textures. Listen to our sounds. Engage us with ALL of your senses and we become closer, more able to help in our oneness.

Do not fear, dear one, we will help the planet ascend. We will help you ascend. We are conscious beings, and deeply loved, deeply loving. Play more with our connection. Train yourself to see and feel our energies.

Let us communicate on ever more clear levels. Our energies are intertwined with yours.

When you feel the power of the seed, of the acorn, that holds the whole tree within, know your own potency. Banish doubt and reclaim yourself. Dance within the grand dance. The magic is real.

[Feelings: Total comfort, peace, beauty, abundance, deep knowing that all is perfect and everything will be okay.]

The Divine Light Invocation Mantra

This strong, beautiful mantra commands protection, purity, and perspective of oneness. I first experienced it at the Yashodra Ashram, in the Kootenay Mountains of British Columbia, Canada. It is a magical, quiet, sacred place on the shores of a lake.

Standing in a round, pure white domed temple that is also a lotus, I raised my arms and chanted this mantra in a circle with perhaps forty others. That evening, on the jewel-green carpet, my sister and I sang sacred songs while snow fell on the lake outside.

THE DIVINE LIGHT INVOCATION

I am created by Divine Light.

I am sustained by Divine Light.

I am protected by Divine Light.

I am surrounded by Divine Light.

I am ever growing into Divine Light.

Give it a try. See how it feels.

What is it like at a whisper?

What does it do when spoken with a commanding voice?

What does it feel like if you resound it silently within?

Integrating the Eighth Initiation

Processing and practicing what you have learned here will take time.

Allow the wisdom, love, truth, and possibilities of light, energy, and consciousness to weave its way into your life in whatever manner is right for you.

Continue to practice the meditations, visualizations, and energy exercises that feel good and call to you.

Do this on a regular basis.

Develop your meditation practice so that it is not only a part of your daily routine, but becomes a delightful adventure into the world of light, energy, and profound alignment with your highest Self.

Go fly with your Dragon!

Be sure to make entries in your Rider's Journal about what you experience in meditation, and write out any variations and visualizations you discover on your own that work for you. This is a very personal practice, and the techniques given here are only the tip of the iceberg of what is possible!

The Ninth Initiation:
Practice

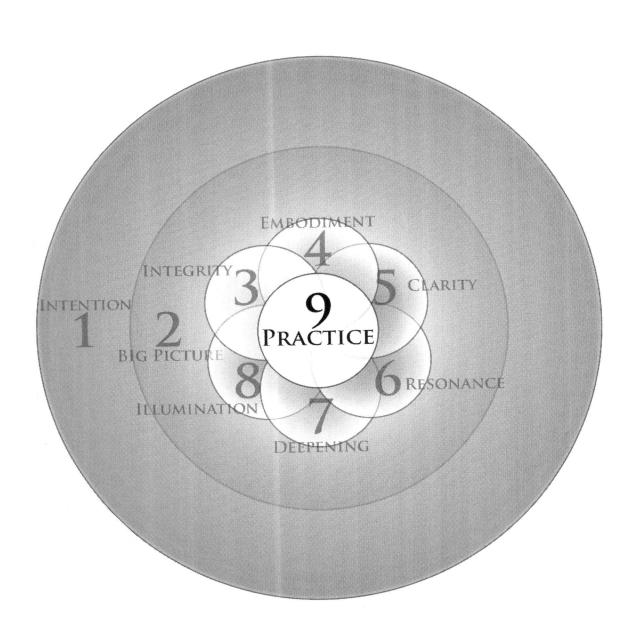

Continuing The Pursuit of Mastery

Congratulations! You've made it this far.

If you choose to accept, you may now step fully into the role of Dragon Rider.

If you have integrated even a portion of this Training into your life—with love, power and wisdom in balance—you have earned this designation.

You are a Dragon Rider.

May your Dragon be a glorious embodiment of Shakti.

And may you ride with wild joy, beloved devotion, and ever expanding ability.

WHAT YOU HAVE LEARNED:

You have learned that a Dragon Rider is one who lives with intention and skill, integrity and devoted service.

You have learned that, first and foremost, you must Know Thyself. When you know your purpose, you can Set Intention and bring meaning to who you are and how you live.

You have learned what it is to look for the beauty in life, and to see the Big Picture.

You have been shown the Empowering Principles of Integrity—the yamas and niyamas. You know why they are crucial, and that they are natural virtues of the heart.

You have been given many practices: ways to align and move, breathe, and expand your capacity in the experience of embodiment.

You know the power of meditation and connecting to Source, as well as weaving what you believe into the way you live.

You understand that resonance and vibration shape all worlds, and that there are ways to attune with specific frequencies, as well as influence those around you.

You have played in the tapestry of philosophy and tasted the nectar of wisdom.

You have been shown ways to work with light and energy, as well as ways to connect with the Masters and Light Beings who are unseen yet ever-present.

THE NEXT STEP IS SIMPLE.

Practice.

Continue your practice in the ways that are best for you. But do not give up. Do not allow the integrity of your practice to crumble, no matter what happens around you or within you.

The way your practice looks will change. And, of course, the constant change of life is forever helping you undergo metamorphosis and transformation.

Know This:

We live in a time when there is so much unknown, so many powers influencing What Is, that life has become quite intense.

Do not let yourself be pulled into the drama of fear.

Hold to the Light. You are the Light.

As a Dragon Rider your choice is to BE Light, to choose Light in every single moment, even as you are affected by the full spectrum of human feelings.

Do not turn away from reality, but choose your focus well.

See the touching moments when tragedy hits.

Look for the heart of Grace in moments of sadness.

Receive the blessing of your breath in full awareness, even when you feel anger.

Always, in every moment, look for the beauty inside yourself and in what you see around you.

Find the good that is the essence of All That Is.

Remember, again and again, who you truly are—a loving, wise, powerful, Divine being.

And, in the ways that call to you, rejoice! Celebrate being alive!

This is the key. This is the point of no return that is celebrated and sought.

For, when you fully embrace this life as a practice of discovering the Divine in each moment, then the whole adventure opens up to you, and magic abounds!

This is how you change the world.

The Heart of Your Dragon

The following meditation was given to me, and to you, from my Dragon. It is a way to realize and experience that the connection you have with this amazingly loving guide can be an intimate and joyful expression of oneness.

You are invited to become one with your Dragon.

Into the Heart of Your Dragon

Sit beautifully and take three deep breaths to center yourself.

Illuminate your connection to the Heart of Earth and Sky with the Pillar of Light.

Feel the beating of your heart.

Now, call to your Dragon. Feel as you are surrounded by this presence of love, wisdom, power, and deep peace.

Notice that your Dragon, at this moment, is enormous! An all-encompassing Divine manifestation that holds you in complete love.

Your Dragon speaks:

Dear one. You are beloved to me.

I come to you in this giant form because, right now, you are the size of my heart.

Exactly the size of my heart.

And so I surround you—enveloping you with light. Cradling you within my heart.

Let us breathe together breath infused with the purest love.

Feel your heart beat and know that I feel it too.

Sit for a moment, and just BE within my heart.

. . . Take your time here . . .

And now, let us FLY together!

As you take a deep breath I spread my wings. We can journey anywhere.

Let us soar, for the simple joy of being together.

Fly with me, beloved.

You are ever within my heart.

Integrating the Ninth Initiation

What do you do now?

Well, in the interest of keeping this book light enough to pack on Excursions, Missions and Adventures, there is a whole world of continued training online.

Visit **www.YogaForDragonRiders.com** to see what's offered by the way of Mastery Courses, Sage School, and the Playground.

Enjoy your own exploration, as I'm sure you will find other avenues and perspectives to integrate with these practices.

Live.

Live fully. Joyfully.

Live in the way that is best for you.

Connect to the essence of power, balanced in wisdom and love. Integrate and deepen.

Apply what you have learned to all of life as you yourself are transformed.

Intertwine layers of you; access the higher vibrations of who you are within the density of the Third Dimension.

Invite your Dragon to be a part of who you are; experience yourself as a being of beauty and power that soars with freedom and sparkles with Light!

Contribute in Your Own Way and Create a Beautiful New World!

The world is changing.

A new age is upon us.

We are on the cusp of a great transition, and it is up to us to give direction and focus; to shape what comes. Those who choose the Light are revered, for they empower the Golden Age we all seek.

In order for harmony to rule, we must choose it. In order for this Earth to be balanced, we must choose it.

You must make this choice yourself. But know that, as you endeavor to live a life dedicated to goodness and aligned with Grace—simply by being your authentic self—you make an immeasurable contribution to what ultimately becomes our world.

The world is changing. It is happening Now. Dragon Riders of great integrity, insight, and illumination are needed! We are very fortunate to count you among them.

May your path be blessed.

Namaste.

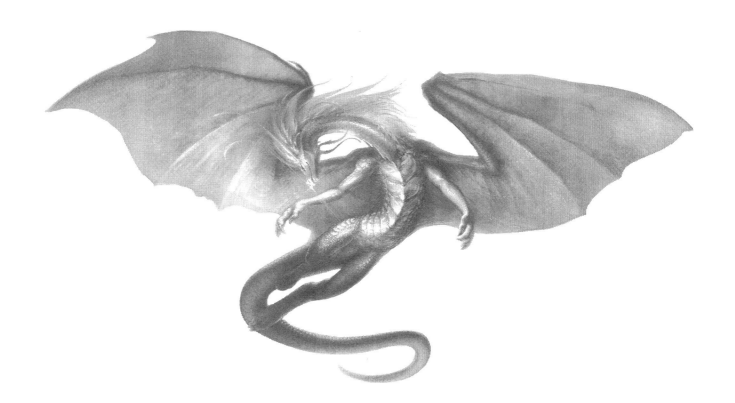

Continuing Studies

Akashic Records

To learn how to read the Akashic Records from Juliette Looye, visit:

www.FengShui-Transformations.com

Suggested Reading

FICTION:

Dragon Rider by Cornelia Funke

Everyone Knows What a Dragon Looks Like by Jay Williams

Illusions by Richard Bach

Lineage of the Codes of Light by Jessie E. Ayani

The Alchemist by Paulo Coelho

The Chronicles of Narnia by C.S. Lewis

The Inheritance Cycle by Christopher Paolini

The Lord of the Rings by J.R.R. Tolkien

The Name of the Wind by Patrick Rothfuss

The Song of the Lioness Quartet (and anything else) by Tamora Pierce

The Ultimate Hitchhiker's Guide by Douglas Adams

NON-FICTION AND SACRED TEXTS:

Autobiography of a Yogi by Paramahansa Yogananda

Be Here Now by Ram Dass

Light on the Yoga Sutras of Patanjali and *Light on Yoga* by B.K.S. Iyengar

Love is in the Earth (great crystal resource) by Melody

Poised for Grace by Douglas Brooks

Relax and Renew by Judith Lasater

The Bhagavad Gita translated by Stephen Mitchell

The Essential Rumi translations by Coleman Barks

The Heart of Yoga by T.K.V. Desikachar

The Source Field Investigations by David Wilcock

The Tao of Pooh by Benjamin Hoff

The Tao Te Ching of Lao Tzu translated by Brian Browne Walker

Wheels of Life by Anodea Judith

Yoga as Medicine by Timothy McCall, M.D.

Online Exploration

For further studies in the realm of yoga, as well as online yoga videos, visit my blog: **www.YogaWithKatrina.com** and also check out my Yoga Radio show.

If you'd like to learn more about meditation and philosophy, subscribe to my free online meditation service at **www.DailyDosesOfDelight.com**.

And, of course, to further your studies as a Dragon Rider, be sure to visit **www.YogaForDragonRiders.com** frequently. The site will continually be expanded with more Training and ways to grow your practice.

To dive into a deeper understanding of the Niralamba Upanishad, take the online course with Christopher Tompkins at **www.Shaivayoga.com/anusara_invocation.html.**

For awesomely inspiring and generally funny tidbits of wisdom, check out **www.Tut.com** and subscribe to the Notes from the Universe.

To shift your idea of the Universe via a radical (and brilliant) approach to physics, visit **www.TheResonanceProject.org** or look up videos of Nassim Haramein. He also does an excellent job of explaining sacred geometry in a way that is relevant and intelligent.

If you want to go beyond conspiracy theories and get researched, documented, well presented information on subjects ranging from the economy to UFOs, get to know the work and blog of David Wilcock at **www.DivineCosmos.com**. You can also watch hours of his online videos that will, very likely, blow your mind.

Gratitude (The Short List)

Life, Nature,
my beloved—Casey Kaldal,
Mom and Dad, my kitties,
Trees, Animals, the Elements,
Ascended Masters, Archangels, the Akashic Records,
Juliette Looye, Antera and Omaran, Scott Marmostein,
Wendy Grono, Carol Bell, Val Theroux, Michelle Morrison,
Tara Findlay, Jen Larsen, Danica Crawford, Elizabeth Beeds
Douglas Brooks, Tony Robbins, Brendon Burchard, Frank Kern,
David Wilcock, Nassim Haramein, All my Facebook friends,
Stars and Earth, The Universe

Every single breath . . .

An incomplete list of amazing yoga teachers who have influenced my life, in deliberately random order:

Shane Perkins, Patrick Creelman, Katie Lane, Elizabeth Rainey, Denise Benitez, Cat McCarthy, Laura Flora, Aaron Lind, Noah Mazé, Sundari, John Friend, Desireé Rumbaugh, Betsey Downing, Michelle Synnestvedt, Elena Brower, Bernadette Birney, Sianna Sherman, Jordan and Martin Kirk, Craig Perkins, Ulla Lundgren, Amy Ippoliti, Lisa Brackenhofer, Angie Edgson, Kristen Cambell, Todd Inouye, Kelly Hass, Gina Minyard, Elissa Gumushel, Marcia Wilson, Tanya Di Valentino and my Yandara family, Katrina Knudsen, Jessica Cristen Pruitt, BJ Galvin, Jenny Sauer-Klein, Rainbeau Mars, the Anusara Kula and the Kula Without Borders . . . and so very many others.

If you know me, and you are part of my Universal Family, you have been a part of my life.

Thank you, each of you, heart to heart.

And to each of my students, who are also my teachers, I bow.

Namaste.

Glossary

ahimsa: the practice of loving kindness, non-violence, non-harming. (uh-HIM-sah)

akasha: space, sky, ether, heaven. (ah-KAH-shuh)

aparigraha: the practice of living simply, non-greed. (uh-pah-ree-GRAH-hah)

asteya: the practice of non-stealing. (ah-STAY-yuh)

bandha: lock or binding. (BAHND-hah)

bhava: feeling. (BHAH-vuh)

brahmacarya: the practice of unconditional love and highest integrity. (brah-muh-CHAR-yah)

dharma: duty; walking your own path. (DHAR-muh)

guru: weighty one; one who brings light to darkness. (GOO-roo)

Ishvara-pranidhana: the practice of deep devotion and joyful surrender. (ISH-wuh-ruh-pruh-need-HAH-nuh)

karma: the cycle of cause and effect. (KAHR-muh)

kundalini: energetic power that rises from the base of the spine to the third eye. (koon-duh-LEE-nee)

lila: divine play. (LEE-lah)

maha: great. (MAH-huh)

mantra: sound in repetition, chanting. (MAHN-truh)

Matrika Shakti: the power of words and sound. (MAH-trih-kuh SHAHK-tee)

metta: Buddhist practice of loving-kindness. (MEHT-tah)

namaste: a greeting, literally "I bow to the Divine in you." (NAH-muh-stay)

niyama: ethical principles for relationship with the self. (NEE-yah-muh)

prana: life force, vital power of life energy. (PRAH-nuh)

pranayama: breathing practices. (prah-nuh-YAH-muh)

samadhi: enlightenment, nirvana. (suh-MAHD-hee)

samskara: habitual pattern; a trench or rut. (sum-SKAH-ruh)

santosha: the practice of deep contentment. (sahn-TOH-shuh)

satya: the practice of truthfulness. (SAHT-yuh)

Savasana: final relaxation in a yoga practice. Also called corpse pose. (sha-VAH-sun-ah)

Shakti: the creative power of the Universe; the Goddess, Divine feminine. (SHAHK-tee)

shanti: peace. (SHAHN-tee)

saucha: the practice of purity. (SHOW-chah)

Shiva: auspiciousness; God, Divine masculine. (SHIV-ah)

svadhyaya: the practice of deep study of the self and yoga. (swahd-HYAH-yuh)

tantra: non-dual philosophic approach to life and yoga; takes the premise that everything, at its essence, is Divine. (TAHN-truh)

tapas: the practice of discipline serving delight. (TAH-puhs)

uttanita: wide open; an expanded view. (oot-TAH-nih-tuh)

yama: ethical principles for relationship with the world around you. (YAH-muh)

yoga: union. (YOH-guh)

About the Author

Katrina Hokule'a Ariel is the only child of two educators who taught her at a very young age to dream big and follow her heart. Her path in life has taken many turns and sometimes convoluted detours, pursuing everything from music and art to motorcycles and snowboarding. Yoga has brought her steadiness and an avenue to expand in so many ways.

Nature has always been Katrina's sanctuary, and some of her best friends are trees—particularly the Live Oaks in New Orleans and the Redwoods in California. She lives in the mountains of British Columbia, Canada (and often elsewhere in the world) with her beloved, Casey, and their two cats.

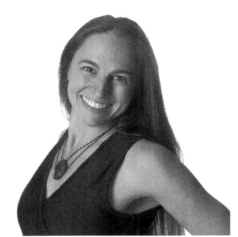

Katrina teaches from the heart, sharing her love of life and joy of creative expression as a contribution of light to the world. She has studied yoga extensively and earned credentials comparable to a Master's Degree in yoga, though she is of the opinion that yoga is something you can spend lifetimes learning. Her vision is to empower and inspire as many people as possible to life fully, in harmony with each other and the Earth.

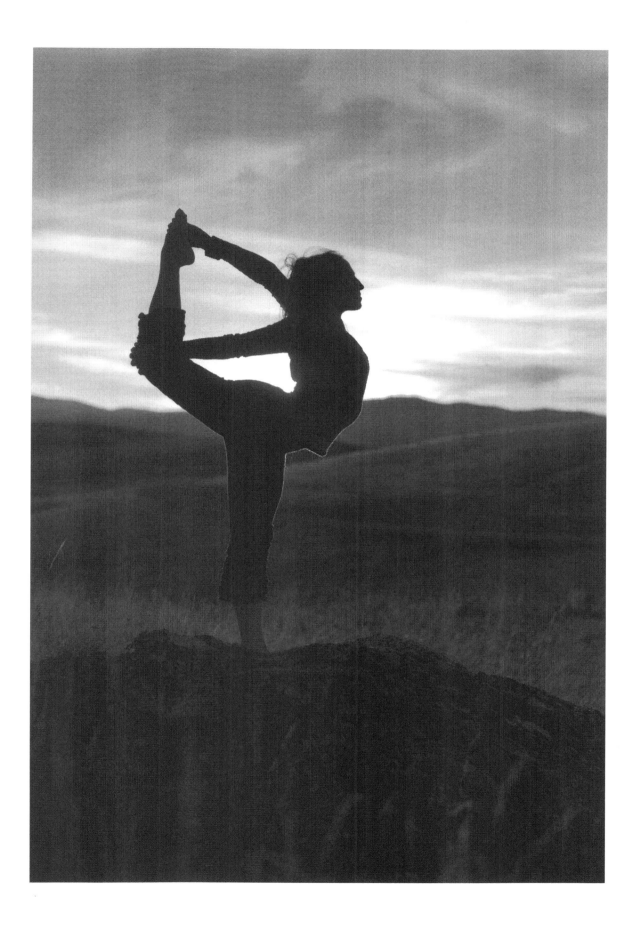

Made in the USA
Charleston, SC
01 August 2012